PRIDE AND JOY

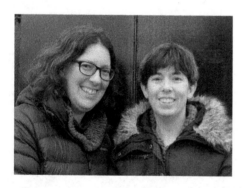

Rachel and Sarah Hagger-Holt are lesbian
parents with two young children. Rachel is
a clinical psychologist and Sarah works in
charity communications.
Together, they have previously written
Living It Out: A survival guide for lesbian,
gay and bisexual Christians, their friends,
families and churches.

PRIDE AND JOY

A GUIDE FOR LESBIAN, GAY, BISEXUAL AND TRANS PARENTS

Sarah and Rachel Hagger-Holt

pinter & martin

Pride and Joy: A guide for lesbian, gay, bisexual and trans parents
First published in the UK by Pinter & Martin Ltd 2017, reprinted 2024
Copyright © Sarah and Rachel Hagger-Holt 2017
ISBN 978-1-78066-420-0
Also available as an ebook
The right of Sarah and Rachel Hagger-Holt to be identified as the authors of this work has been asserted by them in accordance with the Copyright, Designs and Patent Act of 1988
Edited by Emma Grundy Haigh
Index by Helen Bilton
Proofread by Debbie Kennett
British Library Cataloguing-in-Publication Data
A catalogue record for this book is available from the British Library
Pinter & Martin Ltd
Unit 803 Omega Works
4 Roach Road
London E3 2PH
pinterandmartin.com

CONTENTS

INTRODUCTION

The story so far

In the 1970s and 80s, when we both grew up, there were far fewer opportunities for LGBT people to become parents than there are today. Same-sex couples could not adopt jointly, fertility clinics often refused to treat single women or lesbians, and surrogacy was unregulated and inaccessible. And for LGBT families that did exist, it was far riskier to be out. You could lose custody of your children or be exposed by the tabloid press, simply for being an LGBT parent.

In the 1990s, when we both came out, being an LGBT parent was beginning to seem like a possibility. But the reality was still very hard to imagine. LGBT families were still rare and the routes to parenting were not obvious.

Another decade on, and despite not knowing any other LGBT parents, we started our family. And now it seems that LGBT parenting is coming into fashion. Whether they are celebrity chefs, actors, singers, comedians or poets, lesbian, gay, bi and trans people and their kids are now in the public eye. There's even a phrase to describe what's going on: the gayby boom. More and more LGBT people are becoming parents, and living proud and open family lives. There have been radical legal changes which protect same-sex couples with children and enormous strides forward in social attitudes. However, even now, there are distinctive aspects to being an LGBT parent.

On top of all the usual challenges of parenting, LGBT families have to deal with a system and set of assumptions that are not designed for us. We find, even now, there are few role models. Outside certain areas, LGBT families are still unusual. When we talk about our families, we still have to brace ourselves for confused looks, intrusive questions or even hostility.

Why read *Pride and Joy*?

That's why, as LGBT parents ourselves, we think that sharing stories, advice and experiences is so important. We believe that we are stronger together. *Pride and Joy* shares those stories through the voices of more than 70 contributors, of all ages and backgrounds, on a range of parenting topics.

What is *Pride and Joy*?

Pride and Joy is not a manual telling you how to become a parent, or how to be a better one. Instead, it's an invitation to join a conversation. There's plenty of information and advice in these pages, which comes from parents themselves: the people who know first-hand what it's like being an LGBT parent in the UK and Ireland in the 21st century. There are other voices in this conversation too – in particular, the children of LGBT parents, both those who are growing up now and those who are already adults. They won't tell you the path you must follow. But we hope that their stories will spark moments of recognition; that their advice will help you find new solutions to your own dilemmas; and that in sharing some of their laughter and their tears, you will find yourself to be part of a community.

You're invited to listen in, whether you're tentatively wondering about starting a family, your children are hitting the teenage years, or they've flown the nest long ago. We'd also love you to join us if you're a professional working with LGBT families, as a teacher, social worker or midwife, for example, or if you're a friend or family member wanting to support the LGBT parents and their children who are part of your lives.

We hope the conversation will continue away from the pages of *Pride and Joy*. There are now so many ways to meet other LGBT parents – through social media, local groups, or at large-scale events like Pride – and yet many still feel isolated and unsure. Even if you are fortunate enough to have good LGBT friends to share experiences with, the busyness of daily life means that deep conversations are not always possible. There are also some questions which we may not feel comfortable asking those closest to us. We hope the issues, hopes and fears shared in this book will set off new conversations between you, your family and friends.

Who's in *Pride and Joy*?

The biggest challenge in writing *Pride and Joy* has been expressing and exploring the incredible diversity of LGBT families in the UK and Ireland today. It's also been the most fascinating part of this project, as every family's story is full of twists and turns, each unique and touching in different ways. It's been an immense privilege to have been trusted with these stories. It has also exposed the impossibility of making generalisations about the lives and experiences of LGBT families. Contributors' circumstances differ in almost every conceivable way, from where they live to their ethnic backgrounds, ages, abilities and disabilities, political beliefs, attitudes to parenting, jobs, religions and so much more.

Some of the contributors to *Pride and Joy* are single parents, some parent alongside a partner, some are donors, others co-parent with friends. Some have adopted or fostered children, some have children through surrogacy or sperm donation, others had their children in straight relationships before coming out. There is no single type of LGBT parent represented here.

The situation of gay couple Richard and Steven, who spent thousands of pounds and travelled halfway across the world to become parents through surrogacy, is vastly different to that of lesbian mum Poppy, who fell pregnant by accident while still at school. What about Rebecca, who's bi, and her husband, who from the outside look like a straight family; or Katharine, a single woman with a trans history, bringing up two teenage sons by herself; or Scott and Tristan, who adopted their children at a time when LGBT parenting was virtually unknown? All these people, and many more, share their stories in the pages to come. With such diversity, it's inevitable that there will be perspectives and experiences that haven't been fully expressed here, and we apologise for any omissions.

How to read *Pride and Joy*

You can dip in and out of *Pride and Joy*, or you can start at the beginning and read through, or you can follow wherever your own questions or interests lead you. If you want to know more about any of the contributors, simply flick to 'Who's who in *Pride and Joy*' on page 12 to check out who they are. Each chapter ends with 'top tips', written with LGBT parents in mind. However, we hope that all the rest of the stories, experiences and advice will be interesting and relevant, whoever you are.

The first section – 'Starting out' – explores the experiences and expectations that influence attitudes to becoming parents, and the different possible routes to parenthood. If you're interested in starting a family, or want to know more about the adoption process, what it's like to choose a sperm donor, or how to find a surrogate, this is the place to begin. This section raises questions unique to LGBT families, and gives answers that you won't find in mainstream parenting books.

There's far more to parenting than pregnancy, birth or adoption. That's why in the second section – 'Coming out as a family' – we look at what it's like being out as LGBT parents in some familiar settings, including antenatal classes, family gatherings and the school playground. Dip in here if you want to see how the wider world reacts to LGBT families, and to find advice to help with being out and about.

In section three – 'Creating new forms of family' – we reflect on some of the things that make LGBT families different. By opening up new understandings of gender roles, re-examining the nuclear family and showing how significant non-biological relationships are, LGBT families can offer new insights to *all* kinds of families. If you want to wrestle with some of the big questions about what it means to be an LGBT family today, this is the place to begin.

In the final section – 'Who do we think we are?' – we look at questions of identity. If you're wondering how to talk with children about what it means for them to be part of an LGBT family, how to help them deal with change or how to maintain a positive LGBT identity for yourself and your family, then this is the section for you.

Scattered throughout *Pride and Joy* are a number of special features, each of which highlights a particular aspect of LGBT parenting by focusing on a single story. These features bring to life topics as diverse as being a straight ally, choosing not to have children, and how to thrive in a cross-cultural relationship.

The story continues

As LGBT parents, we have good reason to be proud. We are part of a community which has had to struggle to win equal rights and recognition. We can be proud of what we've achieved, and grateful for the efforts of those who came before us. At the same time, we recognise that the struggle still goes on, both here and around the world.

There is great cause to be joyful for those who, because of their sexual orientation or gender identity, never dreamed they would one day be parents. As this book shows, there's much to celebrate about what LGBT families have to offer, whether it's a safe home for a child in need, a challenge to gender stereotypes or a positive role model for a young LGBT person.

This story is our story, and your story. We hope you enjoy *Pride and Joy*. Let us know what you think and join in the story at www.prideandjoybook.wordpress.com or on Twitter @LGBTparentbook

Sarah and Rachel

A word about words

We've used 'LGBT', standing for lesbian, gay, bisexual and trans, as a catch-all term for the families who share their stories in *Pride and Joy*. When we talk about the specific issues faced by gay men, lesbians, bisexual people or people with a trans history, then we refer to this directly. We've also used 'straight' as a shorthand for referring to families with parents who identify as heterosexual, and 'cis' to describe people who have a gender identity that aligns with the one they were assigned at birth. We recognise that both 'LGBT' and 'straight' cover a huge variety of different family shapes and self-definitions. We know that many other acronyms are also widely used, and we do not intend to exclude anyone who identifies more closely with these terms than they do with 'LGBT'. We are also aware that language is powerful, and for times where our language inadvertently denies experiences or leaves a reader feeling silenced, we apologise unreservedly. When quoting people, we have used their own words and their own ways of describing themselves.

WHO'S WHO IN *PRIDE & JOY?*

This book is stuffed with stories, experiences and advice from LGBT families of all shapes, sizes, ages and backgrounds. Without their honesty and their willingness to share their lives with you, Pride and Joy *wouldn't exist. We are enormously grateful to them all.*

You'll hear from many different people in the pages ahead, and we hope their experiences will shed light on your own. They give their perspectives on questions as diverse as how to celebrate Mother's Day, how much genetics matter or how to answer children's questions about sex and relationships. Some people will appear in only one chapter or special feature; others appear many times throughout the book. This section introduces you to everyone you'll meet in the course of reading Pride and Joy.

In some cases, several members of the same family were interviewed. Everyone who is quoted in Pride and Joy *is listed in alphabetical order by first name, and each individual or family has chosen their own words to describe themselves. All contributors' names are shown in italics in the list below. Some have used their own names. Some have chosen pseudonyms. In one case, we have brought together and anonymised the experiences of different contributors into a single composite persona because they did not want to be identifiable.*

Adam is eight years old. His two mums are *Heather* and *Jo* and he has a three-year-old brother.

Ailsa and *Shirley* are a lesbian couple who co-parent their twins with donor-dad Oliver and his partner, Max.

Alan is a gay man who married a woman and they brought up their two children together.

Alison and Hayley say, 'Our family consists of two mummies, our darling son, our crazy dog and our two cats. We love going for walks with our dog, reading, singing and dancing together and making each other laugh.'

Amy and Pally *Marsdunn* are a gay couple with a son, Finlay, aged two.

Andrew and William are a gay couple with an adopted three-year-old son. Follow them on Twitter at @AJPeckett

Barbara is straight and her granddaughter Faye is a lesbian mum.

Ben and *Rich Plummer-Powell* have been married for six years and enjoy being uncles and godparents to many children of family and friends.

Beth and *Marie* are civil partners. They have a two-year-old son.

Bronwen Rees is mum to a 14-year-old daughter.

Bryony is in her twenties, and was brought up by two mums, and her dad.

Carla and Rita are a lesbian couple who have been together for 20 years and married for seven. They adopted two boys, then aged 21 months and three years old, two years ago.

Cathy and her partner, Maz, are a lesbian couple who both have adult children from previous heterosexual marriages. They are now bringing up their 11-year-old granddaughter who lives with them.

Chantelle is 43, a lesbian and a single parent of an eight-year-old girl who was conceived using donor insemination. She says, 'Just to complicate issues further I'm physically disabled and use an electric wheelchair to get around.'

Clare is the lesbian mum of two primary-school-aged children.

Daisy is a lesbian, feminist writer with one biological daughter. She co-parented her daughter alongside her partner's three daughters, and also had three stepchildren. She is close to her grandchildren and her extended family.

David is a gay man living in London who was 47 when he became a sperm donor to lesbian couple *Nicki* and *Rosie* 13 years ago.

Dawn and *Paula* are a lesbian couple who fostered a hard-to-place child on a two-year therapeutic placement.

Dónal Traynor has been with his partner, *Joseph Bowlby*, since 1994. They adopted their two sons, then aged six and five, in the UK in 2011. They now live in rural Ireland.

Felix and *Evan* are a gay male couple with a three-year-old son, who started their family through surrogacy.

Gill Hanscombe is a feminist, lifelong lesbian and author of several books, including *Rocking the Cradle: Lesbian Mothers – A Challenge in Family Living.*

Han (Hannah) Roiter is 22 with lesbian parents.

Hannah and her partner are a lesbian couple who used egg-sharing to conceive their daughter.

Heather and *Jo* are a lesbian couple with an eight-year-old son, *Adam*, and his three-year-old brother, Matthew. The children were conceived with sperm from the same anonymous donor, with Heather the biological mother to one and Jo to the other. Follow them on Twitter at @skylight99

Helen and her partner are a lesbian couple with two children.

Jackie conceived her son, *Jacob*, now in his twenties, using her friend *Paul* as a donor. At that time, she was living with her partner and her partner's young son who had been conceived using anonymous donor sperm. When the boys were two and nine, Jackie's partner died, leaving her a single parent.

Jacob is a bisexual man in his twenties, who was brought up with his older brother by *Jackie*, a single, lesbian mother.

James and Ethan are a gay male couple, currently in the process of being approved as adoptive parents. They blog at www.3years2men1baby.co.uk

James is a gay man who donated sperm so that two friends of his could have children.

Janice is a lesbian adoptive parent of two daughters. She can be found on Twitter at @JaniceFionaBell

Jasmina (Sally) Rush is married to Karl, and has a 21-year-old daughter. She blogs at sallyrush.blogspot.co.uk

Jay and Dee are a lesbian couple with two children from Dee's previous marriage, and an adopted child. They have fostered five children, and currently have one foster child on a long-term placement.

Jenny and Lucy live and work in London and have a boy, aged six, and a girl, aged four. Both were conceived via the same donor egg and donor sperm so they are biological brother and sister.

Jess is the daughter of lesbian parents, and also identifies as a lesbian herself. She tweets at @Silverpasta

Jessica and her partner are lesbian mothers of two daughters, aged ten and eight. They had children with known donor Simon.

Jo and *Heather* are a lesbian couple with an eight-year-old son, *Adam*, and his three-year-old brother, Matthew. The children were conceived with sperm from the same anonymous donor, with Jo the biological mother to one and Heather to the other. Follow them on Twitter at @skylight99

JoJo and Faye have three children between them, and met after their children were born.

Jon is proud to be gay and is hopeful that one day he will be reunited with his daughter.

Justine Smithies is a 43-year-old trans woman married to her wife, Julie. They have two daughters, Morgan (14), who lives at home, and *Samantha* (21), who lives with her partner and two children. Justine can be found on Twitter @JustineSmithies and blogs at justine.smithies.me.uk

Katharine is a trans woman with two sons.

Katie and Jim have two sons, born after sperm donation. Jim has a trans history.

Kim and Diane are a lesbian couple with two children conceived using a donor. They each gave birth to one of their children.

Lea is a pansexual solo parent to a preschooler. She can be found on Twitter at @leahtova

Leila is straight and her niece *Jackie* is a lesbian mum with a bisexual son, *Jacob*.

Lil and *Kaoru* are a Japanese-British couple living in Japan, with two adult children and a one-year-old son. They are both bisexual women.

Lynn Wilson is married to Glenys and they both live in London with one of Lynn's grown-up daughters while the other two children live abroad. Lynn was brought up by a strict and homophobic father so, although she was aware of her sexuality, she entered marriage to a man and had three children before coming out later in life. She has never been happier!

Marie and *Beth* are civil partners. They have a two-year-old son.

Matthew is a gay man and does not have children.

Mel is a lesbian single mum to two daughters.

Mich (non-birth mum) and *Nicola* (birth mum) have an eight-year-old daughter Anna. They don't have an involved father.

Milly is 11 years old, and lives with her two mums, *Nicki* and *Rosie*, and her older brother.

Miriam is a lesbian who co-parents her nine-year-old daughter with her ex-husband, who is bi.

Naomi is pansexual, and married to Mina/Andy, who is gender-fluid. They have one son, Edward. Find them on Twitter at @misty_mina

Nicholas and *Michael* have been together for 11 years and live in London. Their son, Elliot, was born in March 2013 through altruistic surrogacy in the UK.

Nick Mills and *Rory O'Connell* are a gay couple who hope to start their surrogacy journey soon. They would like gestational twins using both partners' sperm with the same egg donor. They blog at www.gaybirthrightuk.com and tweet @GayBirthrightUK

Nicki and *Rosie* are a lesbian couple with two children in secondary school. Nicki gave birth to them both and they were conceived using home insemination with sperm from different known donors, one of whom is *David*. They and their children, *Milly* and her brother, spend time with both donors and their partners on a regular basis.

Paul is a straight man who donated sperm to his lesbian friend *Jackie*. *Jacob* (now in his twenties) was born as a result.

Paula and *Dawn* are a lesbian couple who fostered a hard-to-place child on a two-year therapeutic placement.

Peter Griffin and Louie are a gay male couple starting to explore becoming adoptive parents.

Poppy had her son, now aged five, when she was 16 and still at school. She shares parenting with her ex-boyfriend and lives with her girlfriend, Kelsey.

Rajo and her partner, Varinder, are a lesbian couple who were pregnant at the same time and now have a son and a daughter in secondary school. The children were conceived using anonymous donor sperm from two different donors and were born within ten days of each other.

Ram is a gay man from India, who hopes to become a father. He is currently seeking asylum in the UK.

Rebecca is bisexual, with an opposite sex partner and two small children.

Rich and *Ben Plummer-Powell* have been married for six years and enjoy being uncles and godparents to many children of family and friends.

Richard Westoby and his partner, Steven, are a gay male couple with twins, who started their family through surrogacy. Richard is author of *Our Journey: One Couple's Guide to US Surrogacy.*

Rory O'Connell and *Nick Mills* are a gay couple who hope to start their surrogacy journey soon. They would like gestational twins using both partners' sperm with the same egg donor. They blog at www.gaybirthrightuk.com and tweet @GayBirthrightUK

Rosie and *Nicki* are a lesbian couple with two children in secondary school. Nicki gave birth to them both and they were conceived using home insemination with sperm from different known donors, one of whom is *David*. They and their children *Milly* and her brother spend time with both donors and their partners on a regular basis.

Sally Xerri-Brooks lives in Birmingham with her wife and two-year-old daughter. She can be found on Twitter at @salxerribrooks and she blogs at www.sallyxerribrooks. wordpress.com

Samantha Smithies is the daughter of trans mother *Justine*, aka

Mummy, and Julie, her natal mother.

Sara (birth mother) and Kate (non-birth mother) have an eight-year-old son, Tom, via IVF. They recently separated and are now co-parenting.

Scott and Tristan are a gay male couple who have adopted three sons, now aged 17, 16 and nine years old. Scott is also Senior Regional Manager for Adoption UK, the UK's largest adopter-led Adoption Support Agency and sits on the Department for Education's Adoption Support User Group. Follow their blog at www.gayadoptiondad.blogspot.com or find them on Twitter at @GayAdoptionDad

Shoshana Devora is in her late twenties and was raised by lesbian mums back when it wasn't so common. She blogs about growing up with two mums at mymotherfullfamily. wordpress.com or find her on Twitter @Shoshana_Devora

Shirley and *Ailsa* are a lesbian couple who co-parent their twins with donor-dad Oliver and his partner, Max.

Silvia Melchior is female, currently straight, and married to a man. They have a young child.

Sophie and Nikki are a same-sex couple with a one-year-old daughter. They are the primary parents, but have chosen for the biological father to remain known and involved.

Susie is a stealth transgender woman and 'the other mum' to a teenage girl and her younger almost-teen brother.

Tony is a single gay dad of a teenage son.

Tricia (31) and her partner are a lesbian couple with a two-month-old daughter.

Victoria and Nina *Lawson* are a lesbian couple. Nina gave birth to their three-year-old son using anonymous donor sperm at a clinic.

Yasmin and Lizzie are a lesbian couple, who co-parent their five-year-old daughter with gay male couple Tom and Damian.

Part One
Starting Out

1

THE JOURNEY BEGINS

This chapter explores the experiences and expectations that influence our attitudes towards becoming parents; shares how different people have approached the decision to start a family; and introduces some of the routes that lesbian, gay, bi or trans (LGBT) people can take to become parents.

'Let's start at the very beginning, a very good place to start,' sang Julie Andrews in *The Sound of Music*. And indeed it is. But where *do* we begin? For creating a family doesn't begin with an adoption, a birth or even a conception. It starts much earlier than that: in our own upbringing, in society's ideas of what a parent is or should be, and in the experiences that shape us growing up.

Most of us grew up with heterosexual parents and, regardless of what our families of origin were like, we all grew up surrounded by images of heterosexual families – from children's books to TV soaps to advertisements for gravy granules. Among this sea of straightness, there may have been only one or two, if any, families with openly gay, lesbian, bisexual or trans parents. These early experiences shaped our expectations of what parenthood is or isn't. They formed our impressions of what makes a mother or a father, and our ideas about what is possible for ourselves. If you are LGBT and considering becoming a parent, you'll examine your assumptions about parenthood and will need to decide which to keep, which to reject and which to give a queer twist and claim as your own. There is no clear, well-trodden path to follow.

There are many similarities between families which have parents who identify as LGBT, and those with parents who don't, but there are differences too. Above all is the diversity of ways in which LGBT families can form. In the following chapters, we've separated out these routes to forming a family into five categories: adoption; co-parenting and being or using a known donor; using anonymously donated sperm and/or eggs; surrogacy; or opposite-sex relationships.

'Climb every mountain': Overcoming the doubts

We asked parents who contributed to *Pride and Joy* when they first started thinking about having children. Their answers tended to begin either: '*I always...*' or '*I never...*' or a painful but potentially joyous, combination of the two: '*I always wanted... but never expected...*'

Daisy got married at 21 in the 1950s. She knew then that she was a lesbian, but didn't come out until after her daughter was born. The possibilities open to her and the decisions she made in her teens and twenties were shaped by social norms. '*You were expected to get married, expected to have children. There was no other frame, no alternative idea,*' she says. '*You were considered weird, even in your own family, if you didn't. Any woman who was not married was a spinster, someone odd and looked down on.*'

Twenty years later, at least in some places, not much had changed. Dónal came out in the late 1970s. '*At that time, Ireland was very conservative and male homosexual acts were illegal,*' he explains. '*Part of my coming out process was a period of mourning for the children I would never have. LGBT parenting was almost unheard of. Lesbians who had children from previous heterosexual relationships ran a real risk of losing custody of their children because of their sexuality.*' Much as he wanted children, '*under those circumstances, fatherhood was not an option.*'

At the same time, in England, Jackie was also just coming out and trying to reconcile her desire to have children with the received wisdom that lesbians weren't fit mothers. '*There was never a time when I thought I didn't want children, but along with coming out came the misconstrued idea that it wouldn't be part of the picture for me,*' she remembers. '*In those days, lesbians didn't have children.*' But times were changing, and her experience began to contradict her assumptions. '*I moved*

*down to London in my 30s where it became more and more
apparent that actually lesbians were having children. That's
when I started to think: how am I going to do this?'*

We're all influenced by the attitudes and expectations
around us, but the same expectations can inspire different
responses in different people. Some, like Dónal, campaign
for change in laws and attitudes and live to reap the benefits;
some, like Daisy, do what's expected until the pressure of
conforming becomes so great that they forge a new path; and
some, like Jackie, wait and watch and wonder, until their inner
voice grows stronger than the voices around them.

'I have confidence': Making the decision to start a family

Today, thankfully, more role models exist for LGBT families
than there have ever been. There is less pressure on young
people, whether lesbian, gay, bi, trans, straight or unsure, to
get married young to someone of the opposite sex. Three huge
changes in society in recent decades have shaken up attitudes
towards marriage and family life, not just for LGBT people
but for everyone. It's these changes, accompanied by legal
recognition and protection, which have made it easier for LGBT
people to become parents *and* to live proud and open lives.

The first is the opening out of gender roles and the acceptance
of equal partnership. There are still gender stereotypes and
inequalities, but both partners in a relationship are now likely
to work *and* to contribute to childcare; the assumed female
housewife/male breadwinner split no longer holds true.
Having a family headed by two women or by two men is no
longer unthinkable or economically unviable.

The second is the increasing acceptance and use of assisted
reproduction techniques. From donor sperm to IVF, there are
many ways of having children aside from heterosexual sex, for
both straight and LGBT prospective parents.

The third is that, while homophobia and transphobia
still exist, LGBT people are no longer seen as medically or
psychologically disordered. Being LGBT has become an
identity to be claimed and celebrated, rather than a disease
that needs to be treated.

However, just because we *can* become parents, doesn't

mean that all LGBT people are keen to do so. Some decide that they do not want to bring up children. Others take a long time to work out whether or not it is right for them. Rosie is nine years older than her partner, Nicki, and was 35 when they first met. '*I was certain that I didn't want children,*' she says, looking back. '*I'd been part of lesbian culture for a long time, where having children wasn't something you could even think about.*' Yet, over the course of ten years, Nicki's views changed Rosie's mind. '*I wouldn't say she wore me down, but we did talk about it. But however much we talked, my doubts and anxieties were still there.*' Ultimately, their decade-long relationship meant that Rosie knew it couldn't just be about what she wanted. '*I told Nicki she couldn't wait for me to be really sure, because I never would be, the ball was in her court. I made it clear that I loved her enough that, if this was what she wanted, she should go for it.*' And so Nicki did. The couple now have a son and a daughter, conceived with sperm from two different known donors.

For gay men, routes to parenthood, in particular to becoming full-time primary parents, are much more limited, costly and complicated than they are for lesbians, as Dónal discovered. The dreams of fatherhood which he had abandoned after first coming out, surfaced again 15 years later, when he met his partner, Joseph. They both desperately wanted to have children, but at the time gay couples could not adopt in the UK and Ireland, so they started looking at other options.

'*Some lesbian friends suggested that we donate sperm, but were very vague and avoidant about what role, if any, we'd have with any subsequent children,*' he says. '*It wasn't right for us. We knew that we wanted to parent and not just be fancy "uncles" to our children.*' Once the law changed in the UK to allow gay couples to adopt jointly, Dónal and Joseph saw this as the opportunity to realise their dream. They eventually adopted two sons.

It's not just the practicalities which mean that many gay or bi men in same-sex relationships are less likely to expect to become parents. There is the issue of social expectation. Often, girls are encouraged to play with dolls, to coo over new babies and to help out in caring for younger siblings. Generally, boys are not. This was true for most of us when we were growing up, and as much as we might hope things have changed, in many quarters it continues to be true today. If you're in doubt, just watch the toy ads on children's TV. As recently as the 1980s, parenting was considered 'mother's work'. It's hard not to allow this to influence us when we think about becoming parents ourselves.

Just as there are many LGBT people who don't expect to have children, or who struggle to imagine how it could be possible for them, there are many others who have always expected to become parents. They have embraced that expectation alongside their sexual orientation without seeing any contradiction. *'I've always wanted children,'* says Sara. *'I just assumed it would happen to me. I didn't come out until my early twenties, until I met my partner. When I told my mum, the first thing she said was, "But you'll not be able to have children!" My immediate reaction was, "Well, why not?" I had no idea how, but I didn't see it as a barrier even though I didn't know any lesbian families.'* It was many years from that day to the moment Sara first held her baby son in her arms, but she never doubted that was where she was heading.

'When we'd been together for five years, we started talking about having children,' says Sara. *'I wanted to do it, but my partner wasn't keen. She knew she didn't want to get pregnant or carry a child, whereas I felt it was something I needed to do. I started investigating possibilities and joined some online communities. For a long time this was something I wanted and she didn't. We nearly split up over it.'*

Like Sara, Alison has always wanted children. *'I've always been broody,'* she says. *'From the minute I was first given a doll, to growing up and seeing children around and thinking, I want one of those. I thought it would be through the normal heterosexual journey. I imagined it would happen in the way society expects it to.'* Coming out at 25 and moving in with her girlfriend weeks later didn't derail Alison's plan, it just meant she had to change course a little bit. After exploring other options, she and her partner chose to adopt.

Matthew, who has volunteered and worked in children's services since he was 16, also assumed he would one day become a parent. But he only started thinking about it seriously a few years ago. '*I was in a committed relationship at that time, and I met with a female couple in a same-sex marriage to discuss the idea of co-parenting,*' he says. After initial discussions, he decided not to take this further. '*The main thing that made me decide not to go ahead was the distance of 150 miles between us. I felt that I would either want to be involved in a meaningful way, or not at all. I didn't want my involvement to be tokenistic. My then partner was also less keen than I was, largely for the same reason.*' At this point, Matthew realised he didn't want to try other options for becoming a parent. The time hadn't been right for him in previous years, and it wasn't right now, but for different reasons.

'*I have financial assets, stability, experience and self-awareness now that I didn't have to the same degree a few years ago,*' he reflects. '*However, I also think I have less tolerance and patience now for the demands of small ones. I have become more set in my ways as I have got older and more used to my own space. I enjoy the company of adults, and find long periods of time where conversation is all about the children a little draining! I think I would have been better able to manage physically and emotionally at 29 than 39, but at that point in my life I had less experience, money and job security. I have wondered whether it takes a little longer for some people (me?) to, not grow up as such, or come to terms with something about themselves as a same-sex lover, but to feel fully confident in all that means and to feel they have experienced all they want to before becoming a parent. I haven't regretted this decision since. My dogs are probably a sort of substitute children, like toddlers who never grow up!*'

'A few of my favourite things': Finding, and becoming, role models

Understanding expectations and assumptions – our own, our families' and those we encounter each day in the media and wider culture – is the first step on the road to forming an LGBT family. Because if these expectations say that you can't be a parent because you're LGBT, or that LGBT families are unnatural or don't exist, then they need to shift before you can even begin to imagine creating a proud and happy family.

For some people, these expectations gradually change as they learn more about themselves. For others, there is a defining moment or encounter when they realise that having children is possible for them. When Peter came out at 17, he was supported and affirmed by both family and friends. But his picture of his future as an adult gay man did not include having children. *'When people asked if I wanted children, I would say no. I can't give a clear explanation why,'* he says now. *'I wasn't against being a parent. Was it simply that I could not see how it could happen? Was I just giving the answer that I thought people wanted to hear, or did I genuinely believe it was wrong?'* In his early twenties, Peter started to work with children and families. *'During this time, I started to believe that I could have something to share and I wanted my life to be more than just me. The issue I previously held of being gay and a parent no longer held true.'* Many years later, Peter and his partner are now planning to start their family through adoption.

Tricia, whose partner has recently given birth to their first child, remembers the moment in her life when her expectations shifted and changed. *'Before the age of 22, the areas of my brain labelled "parenting" and "gay" had not yet overlapped,'* she recalls. *'I knew I wanted a family, at some point. I knew I was gay. But I hadn't thought seriously about how the two could work together. I'd never seen any gay families, either in real life or on TV. And I was too busy furtively searching "how lesbians meet each other" through dial-up Internet on the shared family computer as a 16-year-old to look online for positive gay parenting role models.*

'But at 22 I met a lesbian couple who had adopted two sisters. They were so positive about the experience of adopting and what it had meant for them. I looked around their home, brimming with children's drawings and scattered toys; I saw how smiles stretched across the women's faces when I asked them about their children. I also met two gay mums who had written children's story books that acknowledged LGBT families. These encounters started a flickering light in my brain. Ah, I thought, this is A Thing. Happy Gay Families. I didn't know too many happy families full stop, so it was heartening to meet two gay families that seemed to be

thriving. I was instantly won over to the idea.'

Did those families ever know the impact they had on Tricia? Probably not. The stories and experiences of LGBT parents in *Pride and Joy* may have a similar impact on you. They may change, challenge or confirm your expectations of why people become parents and what starting an LGBT family means. It's not just the families who have shared their stories here who are challenging expectations. Everyone living in an LGBT family has an impact on the people around them and their expectations and assumptions, simply by living as honestly and openly as possible. It's a responsibility and it's a joy, even if we never fully know the impact it is having.

In the following chapters, we'll look at the nitty-gritty: the what, who and how of starting a family. We'll hear from people who have started their families in very different ways, as they share some of the difficulties, joys and surprises they encountered along the way. We'll return to their stories and many more in future chapters and see what happens to these families after birth, adoption or family formation.

Top tips

1. **Start with your values.** Your values – whatever they are or however unconsciously they are held – should be your starting point when thinking about how to create your family. No one has exactly the same combination of experiences, beliefs, values and gut feelings as you do, so start by working out what your own attitudes to parenthood are. For example, beliefs about the significance of your child knowing its genetic heritage, or the principle of creating a new life instead of adopting a child in need of a family, will influence the decisions you make. You may have to defend these many times to questioning friends, family members, social workers or medical professionals, so it is a good idea to be clear in your own mind what your values are!

2. **Don't forget the practicalities.** Do you have enough money for a fertility clinic? Are you able to be in the right place at the right time to inseminate with a known donor? Do you have a separate room in your house for an adopted

child? There are various basic questions to consider when you start exploring different parenting options.

3. **Expect the unexpected.** You, your partner or surrogate might get pregnant first time and have to rush into preparations that you thought you'd have months to organise. You might experience many disappointments and pitfalls, and watch years go by before you become a parent. You need to be prepared for it all to go wrong, to lose control of the process and to wonder why you're putting yourself through this. Many people stop and reassess, perhaps several times, on this journey.

4. **Keep a sense of humour.** Because it does feel weird. It feels weird choosing a sperm donor, or a surrogate, or an egg donor, or an adopted child and trying not to feel like you're ordering a takeaway or involved in some kind of dodgy online people-shopping. It feels weird handing over a pot of sperm to a friend or a relative stranger, and it feels weird lying for half an hour with your legs in the air, hoping that gravity will do its work. It feels weird tidying up your house and dressing to impress the adoption social worker, when you know that they'll find out all your secrets anyway in time. It's all a little bit comic. Or at least if you think of it that way, it helps prevent you being overwhelmed by the weirdness and the stress and the panicky feeling of 'are we really doing this?'

5. **Get support.** You and your partner may be totally in tune and united in your quest for a child, with any co-parents 100 per cent with the programme and your extended family offering unconditional support. Or not. It may be that one person in a partnership is less keen than the other on starting a family. It's fine to have a 'lead baby-maker' – the one who's researched different clinics or agencies, joined the online forums, read all the books and bought all the baby clothes – but ultimately, if you are in a couple, this is a joint decision and you'll need to support each other through difficult times. For single parents, extended family and friends are particularly important. You will need to find the right people to mull things over with, and to have a cup of tea with when things get tough.

6. **Do your research.** It's worth checking out the legal implications of any parenting route you go down, so you know what you're getting into. Checking out your employer's maternity/paternity/adoption leave policies is a must for any type of family. For specific LGBT-family-related questions, Stonewall's *Pregnant Pause: A guide for lesbians in getting pregnant* and *Guide for Gay Dads* are brilliant, accessible starting points for parents-to-be in the UK, and can be downloaded for free from their website. If you are unsure, there are lawyers available who specialise in LGBT family law.

LGBT parenting and the law

In the last few decades, there have been radical changes in the law. In case you're struggling to keep up, or can't believe how far we've come, here's a potted history with some key dates.

1975 The group Action for Lesbian Parents is founded after a series of high-profile custody cases result in lesbian parents being denied custody of their children.

1985 The Surrogacy Arrangements Act prohibits the negotiation of surrogacy arrangements on a commercial basis and bans advertising by a prospective surrogate or intended parents.

1988 Section 28 of the Local Government Act comes into force, banning the 'promotion' of homosexuality in schools as a 'normal family relationship'. Although no one is prosecuted under the Act, it leaves many LGBT parents feeling vulnerable to discrimination and schools uncertain whether they can welcome LGBT families, provide positive role models or act against homophobic bullying.

1990 Successful campaign on the Human Embryo Fertilisation and Embryology Bill ensures lesbians continue to have access to fertility services.

2000 Section 28 repealed in Scotland.

2003 Section 28 repealed in England and Wales.

2004 The Gender Recognition Act provides a mechanism for trans people to obtain recognition for all legal purposes in their preferred gender role.

2005 Adoption and fostering by same-sex couples becomes legal in England and Wales. The Adoption and Children Act (passed into law in 2002 and enforced from 2005) allows unmarried couples, including same-sex couples, to apply for joint adoption. It has always been legal for single lesbian or gay people to adopt.

2005 First civil partnerships take place in the UK.

2005 Donor anonymity laws change in the UK. From now on, if someone donates eggs or sperm, any children conceived as a result of that donation will have the right to receive information about the donor once they reach 18.

2007 It becomes unlawful for providers of goods and services in the UK – including adoption and fostering services and schools – to discriminate against people because of their sexual orientation.

2009 Human Fertilisation and Embryology Act comes into force in the UK, giving the right for non-biological mothers, under certain conditions, to be named on their children's birth certificates and to have full legal parental rights and responsibilities. The Act also removes the need for fertility clinics to consider the child's 'need for a father', a requirement which meant many lesbian couples or single women were refused treatment. This is replaced with a requirement to consider the child's need for 'supportive parenting'. Despite this change, barriers can remain for lesbians attempting to access fertility treatment, for example, in some areas you have to have fertility problems in order to be eligible for free treatment.

The same Act states that the birth mother of a child born through a surrogacy arrangement in the UK is always considered the legal parent and, if the surrogate is married or in a civil partnership, her partner or husband will automatically be considered the child's other legal parent. This can only be changed by the court, using a parental order which legally transfers parental responsibility from the surrogate to the intended parents. At this stage, only a heterosexual married couple can apply for a parental order. Single gay men or gay couples, even those in a civil partnership, cannot.

2009   The law changes in Scotland to give same-sex couples equality in adoption and fostering, bringing it into line with England and Wales.

2010   Same-sex couples with 'an enduring relationship' can now apply for a parental order to become the legal parents of a surrogate child. Single people still cannot apply for a parental order for a surrogate child.

2011   First civil partnerships for same-sex couples take place in the Republic of Ireland.

2014   First same-sex marriages take place in the UK.

2015   Intended parents in surrogacy and 'foster to adopt' arrangements are now entitled to adoption leave and pay.

2015   Marriage Act passes in the Republic of Ireland, giving same-sex married couples the same rights as opposite-sex couples, including the provision to apply jointly to be adoptive parents.

(Sources: *The Electronic Irish Statute Book*; *Guide for Gay Dads, Pregnant Pause* and *LGBT History Timeline*, Stonewall; *Information for Unmarried Parents*, Treoir; Press for Change; Surrogacy UK)

2

ADOPTION AND FOSTERING

Same-sex couples in the UK have been able to adopt or foster jointly since 2005. Adoption and fostering have always been possible for single LGBT people. Adoption and fostering agencies now actively call for LGBT people to come forward as prospective parents, and each year more are responding. This chapter explores why some people choose this route to parenthood; shares the joys and challenges they face; and gives advice for potential adoptive parents and foster carers.

A first choice

For mum of two Carla, the decision to adopt was an obvious one, shaped by her own upbringing. '*I am adopted myself,*' she explains. '*So having my own children wasn't something I felt I had to do.*' Carla wouldn't have dismissed having biological children if her partner had wanted it, but they both felt the same way.

The combination of Carla's personal experience as an adopted child and her professional experience as a social worker confirmed this was the right path for her. '*I believe that adoption is as good a route as any to having a family,*' she continues. '*It gave my parents and me a fantastic family life.*' And now she and her partner have the same opportunity to create a loving family life with their two adopted sons. '*For some of my heterosexual friends who've adopted, it was very much a second choice,*' reflects Carla. '*Yet for us this decision was our first choice.*'

As Carla says, many straight couples only consider adoption or fostering once they have found that they cannot have a biological child. Same-sex couples or single LGBT people, for whom having a biological child is less easy or expected, are more likely to make it their first choice.

A long journey

Unlike Carla, Alison and her partner, Hayley, were unsure what to expect when they started investigating adoption. '*We originally looked at adoption, because we knew some friends who had adopted. But it fizzled out after the first enquiry*,' remembers Alison. Despite their initial enthusiasm, they found the questioning from the social workers unsettling and off-putting. It made them realise how much thinking they still had to do. '*They asked lots of questions that we weren't ready to answer, including whether we could take a child who was disabled or with learning disabilities. So we put the idea on the backburner, and got a dog.*'

But it didn't stay on the backburner for long. '*Then we started talking about having a biological child, and looked into egg sharing*,' continues Alison. '*Hayley is older than me and at the time was unhappy at work, so we agreed that if we had a biological child she should have the first one and I'd have one later. We really got into the idea, thinking how amazing it would be see our child growing in her. We started looking for a donor.*'

At that point they came back to earth with a bump. '*We had lots of offers from various men – some close friends, some where it felt a bit forward. Most thought they'd get to have sex with both of us*,' says Alison. '*That was awkward. Then people would start suggesting their friends, asking if we'd want to meet them, or saying, "I know this gay guy..." We looked at using a sperm bank too, but that didn't sit comfortably with us.*'

After considering all the options, they finally returned to the idea of adoption and have recently become proud parents to their one-year-old adopted son. The difficulty of finding a suitable sperm donor did play a part, but it was an emotional experience which swung the decision for them. '*We went on holiday with friends and their six-year-old boy, who they'd had through donor sperm, and we had such a good time*,' Alison recalls. '*We realised we loved him so much and he's not even ours; imagine how much we could love a baby who'd already been born. I started crying, and we knew that we needed to adopt. We realised that our child might exist already, we just needed to arrange to be united.*'

Bronwen also took her time to consider becoming a parent. '*I knew I was gay from a young age and had assumed it wasn't going to be easy to have children*,' she explains. '*I had written off parenthood for a number of years.'* Despite being attracted to the idea of adoption and unsure whether she wanted birth children, Bronwen started by looking for a sperm donor among friends and acquaintances, shortly after successfully recovering from an operation that could have left her infertile.

'*I bought a load of ovulation and pregnancy sticks online and became slightly hysterical about it all,*' she admits now. '*I was checking temperatures daily for ovulation, marking them on a chart and then being disappointed that I hadn't ovulated, even on one occasion discovering I had used a pregnancy test not an ovulation test to try to check this out! It was all a bit of a palaver. I quickly became bored of the endless checking and charting.*'

Bronwen made contact with one potential donor, but it came to nothing. That's when the penny dropped and she realised that she wanted to adopt. '*I would love to say I was bitterly disappointed,*' says Bronwen. '*But my heart leapt for joy when I realised I could pursue a dream of adopting instead! I had long had dreams of adoption or fostering (possibly over-romanticised about saving little orphan Annies…) and once I had decided, with a sense of relief, that giving birth to a child wasn't going to happen, I was keen to adopt an older child.*'

Choosing to adopt an older child, rather than giving birth to and caring for a baby, allowed Bronwen to be the kind of parent she wanted to be. She felt strongly about a child's need for a stay-at-home parent, but knew that, as a working single parent, she couldn't be around all the time. However, her working hours as a teacher meant that she could be there for an older child who was already in school. In fact, she felt she could go even further: '*I felt I could take on two children, as being a teacher I am used to working with more than one child on a daily basis,*' she says with a smile. '*In reality, I adopted one – and she is more than enough at the moment!*'

A way of giving back

When Jay and her partner, Dee, began fostering, they already had two children from Dee's previous marriage. Both worked supporting people with learning disabilities or mental health issues, and this sparked their interest in fostering children with disabilities or communication problems. Jay explains, '*In working with adults, I started to wonder what would happen if you caught someone early, before they ended up with deep problems or in a secure unit. Could you make a difference and stop them getting to crisis point? So we started toying with the idea of fostering. Dee was always passionate about it, and I knew I didn't want to carry a child myself.*

Fostering appealed to Dee and Jay because they knew they had something to offer to a child in need of a secure, loving home, but first they had to make sure the rest of the family was on board. It had to be a joint decision. *'When our son moved out, we had a spare room and were able to think seriously about fostering,'* says Jay. *'Our daughter was still at school and lived at home, but worked weekends. They were both very supportive of our plans to foster. It would never have worked in a million years if they weren't up for it.'*

Over the years, Jay and Dee have offered respite care for other foster families, and have fostered five children, including their long-term foster daughter. They have also gone on to adopt, a situation they hadn't expected or planned for. *'Our son came to us at eight months as an emergency placement,'* continues Jay. *'He was supposed to stay six months max. We ensured that he saw his birth parents and he was supposed to return to them, but unfortunately their circumstances meant that never happened.'* It was time for another family decision. *'We spoke with our family about whether to adopt him. We all said, "Let's do it," and put our names forward. So did others from the birth family, but we were the most suitable candidates. The adoption went through, but it was a long and drawn-out process: he was three years old when we finally adopted him.'*

Jay's fostered and adopted children have brought her a great deal of joy, as well as heartache. Fostering is something she believes can be intensely rewarding, for both parents and children. *'When you see someone who is so damaged when they come to you become productive and engaging, then you know you've done your job. It can take a long time and a lot of tears. It's a way of giving back. If no one did this, it would be such a sad society to live in. I believe each kid will one day pay it forward. I'd say to anyone thinking about fostering, do it. You give a child a home and, one day, you can watch them fly.'*

A joy and a duty

Ethan and James are a gay couple just beginning their journey to parenthood. Once they had accepted that their desire to become fathers was stronger than their fear of what society might think about two gay men having children, adoption was the logical choice. '*We'd always felt very strongly that, were we ever to become parents, we'd do it through adoption, as there are already so many children on the planet in need of loving, safe homes,*' explains Ethan. But they weren't expecting the emotional response that came as they snuck into an adoption information evening late and shuffled into back row seats.

Ethan explains what happened that night: '*What struck me immediately was that we were the youngest couple by about a decade and were also the only interracial couple. But then we noticed there was another gay couple, a lesbian couple, single adopters – a whole range of people.*

'*The session went through the whole adoption process, from timescales to police checks. Before then, it had never really occurred to me what kind of children would be up for adoption, but it soon became clear that these children potentially have significant trauma, emotional damage, disruption, developmental delay and even disabilities and long-term illnesses. In short, they've been through a lot of crap before ending up in care and in need of new, loving families. It was a concept that had previously escaped me. I'd imagined we'd adopt a perfect, beautiful, healthy child that just happened to need new parents. But hearing about all the possible complications that these kids might come with, I couldn't help but feel totally overcome with emotion – I was now even more sure than ever that this was what we were supposed to do. Maybe it sounds iffy, but I felt a strong sense of "duty". James and I are only very near the beginning of our journey and already adoption has consumed me in a way that I wasn't expecting.*'

A dream come true

It's only just over a decade since the law in the UK changed to allow gay couples to adopt jointly, meaning that James and Ethan can take their first steps towards becoming adoptive parents. In this short time, adoption has gone from being an impossible dream for a same-sex couple to pursue, to a well-trodden path to follow.

Scott and Tris have two adopted sons, who are now approaching adulthood themselves. When they first got together, they would never have believed this would be possible. They knew they wanted to become parents, yet did not think a gay male couple could adopt children. They tentatively wondered whether fostering could be an option. Scott explains, *'Tris was driving home when a radio advert came on asking for foster carers urgently. We phoned the number advertised and crossed our fingers. To our relief, the person on the end of the phone was gay, and he was so excited that a gay couple had rung as a result of his advert! He explained that there had been changes to UK law, which meant that fostering and adoption were now open to anyone.'*

After a long initial meeting with their social worker, Scott and Tris were excited, daunted and desperate to hear whether she had recommended that they continue. *'We checked the post every day – even the next morning! Then, there it was, what we had been waiting for. Tris opened the letter, as I couldn't handle the thought of rejection. A big smile appeared after he read the three pages. We had been invited on to the Prepare to Foster course with a view to taking our application further! Yippee!'* But that wasn't all. *'We read on a little more – "However..." – uh oh! – "...I would also recommend that Scott and Tris look into adoption, rather than fostering, as I could foresee problems when children were reunited with their families, or placed in an adoptive placement" – OH MY GOD!!! Was she saying we can adopt children? Yes, she was! Even the suggestion of adoption just blew us away.'*

Scott and Tris were in the right place at the right time, coming forward just as the law was changing to enable same-sex couples to adopt. Although there were many delays and obstacles before they finally created their family, just a few years earlier it would not have been possible at all. All they had heard about gay people adopting were sensational and disapproving stories in the media; they even worried that tabloid journalists might turn up on their doorstep. And yet, their positivity and perseverance meant that they became the first same-sex couple to be approved as adopters in their local authority.

Five things you should know

1. **Your sexual orientation shouldn't matter.** To apply to become a foster carer or an adoptive parent, all you need is to be over 21 years old and have a spare room. That's it. Being lesbian, gay, bi, trans, single or in a couple should have nothing to do with whether you are judged suitable – or not – to foster or adopt.

2. **More and more LGBT people are adopting and fostering.** The number is rising each year. For some agencies, up to 10% of their adopters are LGBT. Because there are fewer adopters with a trans history, some agencies may not have experience of this, although like LGB adopters, potential trans adopters are legally protected from discrimination.

3. **You can choose your agency.** Some adoption and fostering agencies are run by local authorities, others are (voluntary) agencies. You don't have to go to your own local authority. So if you feel uncomfortable with a particular agency because of how they treat you as an LGBT person or for any other reason, there are plenty of other options. You can ask other LGBT parents or prospective parents for advice and recommendations.

4. **Your family will grow.** Of course it will, you are adding a child or children to it! In the case of adoption, after living with you for several weeks, the adoption will be finalised by court order and you will become legal parents. It's a momentous occasion and many families choose to celebrate their Adoption Day each year. However, even after adoption, your child may continue to have some contact with their birth family, perhaps through visits or messages. Even if there is no, or very limited, contact, you will still need to be ready to talk to your child openly about their birth family.

5. **Getting support is crucial.** After a long period of training, reflection and assessment, a panel will decide whether you are suitable to adopt or foster. It can then take months or years before you are matched with a particular child and begin a series of introductions. It's a long process of ups and downs, raised hopes, difficult decisions, disappointments and delays. Getting practical and emotional support, both as you go through the process and once your child joins your family, is vital. (*Source*: First4Adoption)

3

SPERM BANKS AND FERTILITY CLINICS

For a woman in a same-sex relationship, or for a cis woman whose partner is a transman, the first obstacle to getting pregnant is finding the sperm needed to conceive. Many solve this problem by using a sperm bank and a fertility clinic for insemination, a procedure known as IUI; or for fertility treatment, such as IVF. In this chapter, those who've chosen this route explain why they did so; and share the ups and downs of the process, including struggles with infertility and what it's like to choose a donor.

Being sole parents

Rajo and her partner, Varinder, thought that using anonymous donor sperm would be clear and simple. It was their first choice. Compared to trying to find a friend or acquaintance to donate sperm, using a sperm bank to select an anonymous donor made it very clear what their roles would be. '*Rather than going to someone we knew or through the lesbian and gay community to find a known donor, Varinder and I wanted to be sole parents,*' says Rajo firmly. '*We didn't want any complications, just a child, that's it, no complex relationship or issues.*'

Using a sperm bank enabled them to make deliberate choices about their children's genetic heritage which might have been difficult when looking for a known donor. Rajo and Varinder both got pregnant at the same clinic in the same month, using sperm from different anonymous donors. '*I wanted a Pakistani donor to reflect part of my identity,*' Rajo explains. '*My partner for the same reasons wanted one from India.*' They were glad to be able to make this choice, but other elements of the process of choosing a donor made them uncomfortable: '*We had so much choice. Height, weight, eye colour, even IQ, you could choose exactly what you wanted, but it felt wrong to be so specific.*'

Choosing a donor

Unlike Rajo and Varinder, lesbian couple Marie and Beth did not plan to start their family using anonymous donor sperm. In fact, it took many years of discussion, exploring other options and wrestling with ethical concerns before they made their decision. '*After I came out, I always assumed I would adopt,*' explains Marie. '*I preferred that idea because then my partner and I would both have the same genetic relationship to our child. I also knew it would be easier for my parents to accept. I got the feeling from my mum that it was more ethical to adopt, rather than to find a market-based solution to the need for sperm.*' But Beth didn't want to pursue adoption. '*There was already so much about having children that was out of our control,*' Beth explains. '*It felt too vulnerable for it to be left for social workers to decide if we could have a family.*'

They were both keen to find a known donor whom they could trust, rather than entering into a commercial relationship. This was the route they pursued initially, but it didn't work out. '*We didn't have a known donor because the people we asked said no,*' says Marie bluntly. '*It was very painful. We asked two couples we knew – one gay, one straight. We couldn't come to an agreement about keeping the donor's identity a secret. It could be okay if the donor was anonymous to us, but not if we knew and our child didn't. That would be keeping secrets.*'

'*Then we thought, once you've been through the list of people you know and trust, and start looking at people you only know through other people, then you're taking a gamble anyway,*' continues Beth. So, in the end, they chose to use a sperm bank, feeling it was the best choice in spite of their doubts. The process of selecting a donor did not make them feel more at ease with their decision. '*It was surreal,*' says Beth. '*It felt very commercial – you pay more money to see enhanced profiles, a bit like on Spotify. In the end, it came down to two: one who looked more like me and one who looked more like Marie.*'

'*We chose the one who looked more like me,*' continues Marie. '*It sounds terrible but his grades were higher! The profile said his parents had the same profession as mine, and we seemed to share the same faith and values.*'

Beth and Marie are not alone in struggling to make such an important choice with such limited information. Katie, who needed donor sperm to conceive because her partner, Jim, has a trans history, felt it was like a bizarre kind of lottery. *'I remember being given the barest of details over the phone by the clinic,'* she says. *'"Donor number 57 is 5'8" tall, medium build with dark hair and proven fertility. Donor number 73 is 5'10" with fair hair and blue eyes." It felt a bit like choosing a Chinese takeaway.'* Like Marie and Beth, they had to allow something to be the deciding factor: *'In the end we went for the shortest donor on offer – because Jim's family are all short.'* Despite their uneasiness with parts of the process, Katie and Jim are deeply grateful to the unknown man who enabled them to give birth to their two sons.

Others, like Victoria and her partner, take the strangeness of the process in their stride. *'I'm quite shallow,'* Victoria admits cheerfully. *'I looked at choosing our donor based on whether they were hot. I thought, If I was in All Bar One in my straight days, would this be someone I would find attractive? I also wanted someone who was honest in his statement – no nonsense about doing this to help out women. If someone said he was doing it for the money, there's a degree of integrity in that.'* Her partner had a more practical approach: *'She was more interested in whether they had a clean medical history, but in the end we agreed on the same guy. Everyone we know who's done this has actually found it quite easy to choose, the right person has jumped out at them.'*

Try, try and try again

The decision to use a fertility clinic is not necessarily an indication of fertility problems for lesbians or female partners of transmen. This choice has less to do with their own ability to conceive, and more to do with getting access to medically screened donated sperm in a safe and legal environment. So when some women fail to get pregnant or miscarry despite repeated inseminations, it can come as a shock. It did for lesbian mum Jo. *'Before the treatment began I worried about all kinds of things, but I didn't worry about getting pregnant,'* she reflects now. *'I thought with two women it must mean double chance.*' But women in this situation are just as likely to have difficulty conceiving as the general population.

Jo explains the difficulties that she and her partner, Heather, faced: '*Heather tried a couple of times with scans and limited medications, then more full-on with hormonal treatment. Each time, I felt sure the insemination would result in pregnancy.*' But after a disappointing two years, they stepped up the treatment from simple insemination to IVF. Their first cycle was NHS funded, and it failed.

'*Suddenly the emotional stakes were much higher,*' says Jo. '*Heather responded well to medication and acupuncture on the second attempt and had 30 eggs taken – I believed that this meant successful treatment for sure! We made the rookie error of naming the two embryos, so when there was no pregnancy it felt like actual children had been lost. It was devastating.*'

Despite the trauma and tears, the increasing costs and the fear that they would never get pregnant, they could still see a funny side to the process. They were now paying for IVF themselves, and the drugs and the donated sperm were delivered direct to their home. Jo remembers hoping the neighbours didn't spot the tank of frozen sperm – with a large sign on the side reading, 'LIVE HUMAN SEMEN' – being delivered to their door. '*The first tank went missing en route,*' she recalls. '*Heather chased round after the delivery van trying to locate it in time to prevent the sperm defrosting and dying. I had a strange notion that it would be accidentally left at McDonald's and get put into a milkshake. There'd be some newspaper headline saying, "Lady Goes for Burger and Comes Out with Bun in the Oven!"*'

Several rounds of gruelling IVF followed, each time feeling like a bigger let down than the last. Eventually they agreed to give it one last try: '*Imagine my surprise and delight to find it had worked! So began eight and a half months of roller coaster hell, culminating in our son being born nearly six weeks early and needing tube feeding in Special Care.*' Despite everything, they had become parents.

Three years later, they started thinking about having another child, '*Given Heather's difficult pregnancy, we agreed that I should be in the hot seat this time!*' says Jo. Two years and four attempts later, she was pregnant with their second son. *'Was it worth the trouble we went through? Definitely,'* says Jo. *'Would I do it again? Not a chance.'*

There is no guarantee it will work, especially for women in their late 30s or early 40s. This brings prospective parents face-to-face with the question of how far they are prepared to go to become parents. *'I started to want to be a parent in my 30s,'* reflects Jenny. *'But at the time I was with a woman who didn't want to have children. I finished that relationship, and decided to make my next relationship with a woman who did.'* Lucy was definitely in this category. By the time they met, she was already actively pursuing her dream of becoming a parent, using sperm from an anonymous donor. But Lucy had been pregnant three times, and had had three miscarriages. Both she and Jenny were now in their 40s so, while having children was something they both wanted, it looked increasingly unlikely to happen. That is, unless they considered not just using donor sperm, but donor eggs as well.

This was a more complex decision, as it meant neither of them would have a genetic connection to their children, but, as Jenny explains, *'In the end this was the only option available to us, that enabled Lucy to carry and give birth to a child. So that's what we did. Much to our delight it took first time.'*

Using donor eggs was not their first choice but it meant that, despite their struggles with infertility, Lucy was able to be the birth mother to their two children: a connection they both saw as important. Their only regret is that they know so little about the sperm and egg donors who enabled them to create their family: *'We sent photos of us both to the clinic so they could match us a little bit, but we know very little detail about the donors. In the country we went to, it's totally anonymous, there's no possibility of getting in touch. We only have basic details. That was really sad. We would have loved to have known more about them. We went abroad because at that time the waiting time for egg donation in this country was simply too long.'*

However, not all women who consider using donor eggs, ultimately decide that this is right for them. Sara always wanted a big family. *'I'm the eldest of four. Having a family meant children, not one child,'* she explains. She and her partner had their first child through IVF with donor sperm when Sara was 36. But she was approaching 40 by the time they started trying again. She continues, '*For various reasons, including the hideous lack of sleep, we postponed trying for another baby. We started IVF again using sperm from the same donor, but the cycle failed and the clinic said we needed donor eggs too. We didn't feel right taking that route; we wanted a full sibling for our son, or nothing. I did so much grieving after the failed cycle that I'd come to terms with the fact we'd probably never give our son a sibling. Now when I see friends with their second or third child, I often count my blessings that we have only one. My son does say that he wishes for a sister, and when I see him with his cousins I wonder, but it is what it is and it has worked out.*'

Unexpected fertility issues can be devastating, and, as Victoria relays, can have consequences on a couple's relationship. Victoria, whose son was conceived after fertility problems, cautions any couple to think carefully before embarking on IVF. '*You need to be 150% certain of your relationship,*' she warns. '*When a woman starts down the process of IVF, it can't be reversed. She's not going to say, "Oh well, it didn't work so we'll stop." It can completely wreck you. It's hard work doing IVF and you need to be certain it's the right thing, especially if you're short of cash.*' Although the experiences in this chapter are of people who succeeded in getting pregnant, many don't, even after several rounds of IVF. Some make the difficult decision to stop treatment, especially if it is threatening their health or their relationship.

Katie and Jim also took several IVF attempts before getting pregnant. '*Once we found the clinic, our journey was more about infertility than about Jim being trans,*' says Katie. '*Becoming parents was difficult and, in the end, expensive. Was that because one of us was trans? Yes and no – in some ways more of the pain came from the difficulties I had conceiving (despite guaranteed A1 quality sperm!). But perhaps for us as a couple it was helpful that we both carried some responsibility. I spent the whole pregnancy convinced that something would go wrong – but, although my son's birth was difficult, both he and I were fine. I will always remember the amazing feeling of holding him in my arms for the first time.*'

Five things you should know

1. **This route to parenting is becoming mainstream.** Fertility clinics and sperm banks in the UK became more accessible for lesbians in 2009, when a change in the law meant clinics were no longer required to consider a child's need for a father before offering fertility treatment. This has also meant that more single, straight woman are turning to sperm banks to help start a family. As a greater number and more diverse range of people choose this option, it has become more socially acceptable. From billboard ads to soap opera storylines to large-scale alternative parenting events, this route is becoming widespread and commercially successful, and attractive for LGBT prospective parents.

2. **The non-biological parent is a legal parent too.** If you are a couple who use donor sperm, both of you can be named on the birth certificate and be legal parents. It doesn't matter if you're in a civil partnership, if you're married, or not, you just have to complete a form at the clinic.

3. **It's not just one decision.** You will face many decisions on your path to parenthood. Which clinic to choose. Which donor to choose. Which form of treatment to go for: simple insemination (IUI), with or without additional drugs, or IVF where the egg is fertilised outside the body and then transferred. Whether to carry on with fertility treatment after a failed cycle. Whether to buy and store extra sperm for a future sibling, and how much sperm to get. There are events, information sessions run by fertility clinics, and a wealth of experience and advice on online forums and websites, all of which can help you make informed choices. However, ultimately you have to make the best decisions you can for your family, regardless of what anyone else says you should or shouldn't do.

4. **You will need determination.** Many LGBT prospective parents find IVF a difficult experience that places strain on their relationships, their well-being and their finances. The appointments and tests are time-consuming and often require travel and time off work. Some fertility treatment is available on the NHS, but not all, so it can be costly.

Other parents insist that, although it can be difficult, if you approach the experience with a positive attitude, there is nothing to be worried about. It's a means to an end and is all worth it. In fact, if you trust the clinic and the staff to have your best interests at heart, it can be reassuring to know that their experience can help you with any legal or medical issues that you face.

5. **Your children may be able to trace the donor.** If you use sperm or eggs from a UK donor, your child will have the right to trace the donor when they are 18. This legal provision has led to a sharp decline in the number of UK sperm donors in recent years. With imported sperm, or treatment at a clinic overseas, your child may not be able to find out who the donor was. However, Internet searches and message boards have enabled some LGBT parents or their children to identify their sperm donor. For families who are interested in knowing genetic relatives of their children, there are thriving online and real-life communities of half-siblings conceived via donor sperm, known as 'diblings'.

4

SURROGACY

Many gay men who want to be primary parents choose surrogacy, in the UK or the US, to start a family. This route can be complicated – finding a woman willing to carry your child, and often a separate egg donor too – and it can be expensive. But it has enabled many to fulfil their dreams of parenthood and created hundreds of new families. This chapter explodes some of the myths about surrogacy; and hears how and why parents choose this route.

Making it real

Nicholas and Michael are a British-American couple, living in the UK. Nicholas was always interested in having children, but says, '*I always assumed it wasn't possible to be a parent. I met Michael in 2005. At that time even adoption was not really a possibility for us as a gay couple. I remember having conversations with other gay people years before. I said I thought I could have children and someone else told me not only that it wasn't good for gay people to have children, but that it was actually wrong.*' However, Michael comes from the States, where there is a longer history of surrogacy, and so had a very different approach. As Nicholas sums it up: '*His attitude is: "if you want it, you can get it", but, being British, perhaps I'm more accepting of my lot.*'

Even though Michael was aware of surrogacy as an option, neither he nor Nicholas knew what it would involve or how to get started. At first, they considered going back to the US or to another country, but ultimately they didn't feel comfortable about the possible exploitation of surrogates in some parts of the world. They didn't know anyone else who'd used surrogacy, so they didn't know what to expect when they stared to explore the options available in the UK. '*When we sent the first email to the gay contact at Surrogacy UK, we didn't hear back for three weeks,*' remembers Michael. '*When they replied, they said,*

"*Sorry, the day you wrote was the day our daughter was born!*" It was a lovely personal reply. They were the first gay couple we knew in the UK who had children.'

The idea was starting to take shape, but it wasn't until Nicholas and Michael plucked up the courage to go to a conference for intended parents and surrogates that it started to feel real. '*We were trembling in the car park outside. We were a young gay couple who didn't know any other gay families,*' continues Michael. '*We went in to find more than 100 people and a flock of children running around, looking happy and well-adjusted. It was a transformational moment. It went from a wonderful, hyper-fictional idea to something in-your-face, showing it works, it happens! It had a wonderful immediate impact on us.*'

After that first conference, it all moved quickly. After three months of visits and tests they joined Surrogacy UK as full members, which gave them access to online message boards and socials where they could informally meet potential surrogates. '*That stage was so emotionally and mentally demanding,*' recalls Michael. '*We were on trains for days, going to socials as frequently as we could. They were usually somewhere like a pub with a play area or a tourist attraction. We went to all sorts of places and had a wonderful time. It was a bit like speed dating: you are yourself, but you project the best version of yourself. Your hopes and dreams rest on this being a success. Then there's the unavoidable analysis on the way home: did we like anyone? Did they like us? It was bizarre.*'

Despite the stress involved, Michael and Nicholas found that this process helped to strengthen their relationship and their determination to become parents. '*If your relationship is really solid, it can be wonderful for you as a couple. You hold each other up and reassure each other that you did come off well,*' explains Michael. '*We kept on going out there, meeting people "naturally", waiting to find that spark. We joined in December, and met Sarah, our surrogate, in March. We did not have to find an egg donor as well, so it was relatively quick.*' Four years later, they have a son.

Early on in the process, the couple decided to keep an open mind about whether to opt for 'gestational surrogacy', where they would need to find an egg donor and embark on IVF at a clinic, or 'genetic surrogacy', where the surrogate uses her own eggs and can inseminate at home. Nicholas explains their very pragmatic reasons, *"We wanted to be in a position where we were ready to go with whatever suited the surrogate mother, whether that was IVF with donor eggs or 'straight' surrogacy. It feels like this was atypical, many other couples had a stronger sense of which route."* In the end, they opted for genetic surrogacy and home insemination.

Making connections

Felix and Evan, whose son is now nearly three, ended up developing a successful, long-term relationship with the woman who bore their child. *'It needs to be a relationship based on trust and how you get on with each other,'* explains Felix. *'I believe you need to meet first before deciding to go ahead, rather than the relationship being determined by a third party. It was probably a bit slower, but based on our experience we have become unbelievably pro this way of doing things, although we know other people may do it differently. It's not just finding someone who can meet your needs and then when you're done, you're done. There is a strong concept of lifelong friendship at the heart of it.'*

He acknowledges that with any relationship comes a risk, but it was one that he and Evan were willing to take: *'It is a risk to make a lifelong relationship with a surrogate, knowing it could lead to pain and not knowing how it will pan out. But I feel much more comfortable knowing the woman, rather than trusting to an intermediary.'*

Like many other couples, Felix and Evan knew next to nothing about surrogacy when they started the process in the UK, and were initially daunted by the prospect of meeting – and trying to impress – potential surrogates. *'The story is that women who have struggled to have their own children become surrogates to "help a woman like them". So we wondered whether they would be interested in us,'* says Felix. *'We're just some guys who want a child. However it turned out it was more emotionally straightforward that way. There aren't the same jealousy issues. If you're a straight woman who can't conceive and you're using a woman who can, you will see another woman carrying the child that you want to carry. It's very different with two guys who know they never would be able to carry a child themselves.'*

They found a woman they clicked with, spending months getting to know her and her husband. They were just about to start IVF when a phone call came. *'She called us up and said she was 10 weeks pregnant,'* says Felix. *'We thought, Oh fuck, what do we do now? This was where being part of the organisation really helped. We hadn't realised before that the surrogates were a "pack" – in the nicest possible way – they were very close and talked to each other. We thought the aim was to find a surrogate you liked and who liked you, but really it was to get the general surrogacy mass to accept you as a good, decent couple who they wanted to help. So the call went out: we need to help these guys. A few weeks later we heard from Danielle. She's a single mum with four kids. In many ways similar to us, in many ways different. She is phenomenal.'*

To the outsider, surrogacy can seem the most medicalised and complicated route to starting a family, the stuff of science fiction, not everyday life. But it is an approach that can be founded on a network of relationships, with human contact and cooperation at its heart.

'When you go back into the mindset of someone first approaching it, it can seem scary and unreal,' says Evan. *'You need to recruit a team of people – the surrogate, the egg donor, their husbands or families – there's a whole legal process. It can seem vast and daunting. But now we're in the relationship, we can see it's the best thing we've ever done. Danielle feels that way too. You can ask why surrogates do it. Pregnancy's awful. But to create a new life, to create a family; when you look back and think what's special about your life, this has got to come top of the list.'*

Making the choice

Nick and Rory spent their first date, a picnic in the park, talking non-stop about anything and everything, including sharing their views on fatherhood and family with each other. *'One of the conversations that came up was our desire to be fathers and to one day have a family of our own,'* remembers Nick. *'That's something that has persisted in our conversations and aspirations ever since.'* Since moving in together, their desire to start their family has grown, partly inspired by the network of people around them. *'We have stumbled upon an amazing community of friends,'* they explain. *'One constant in our community is kids, who drop in and out on a regular basis to impart news, entertain our dogs, cajole sweets, or all three.'*

However, surrogacy was not an obvious first choice. It's still unusual enough to attract questions and raised eyebrows, and expensive enough to be out of reach for many people. Rory and Nick found that people assumed that they would first look into adoption, implying that trying to have biological children was unnecessary and indulgent. *'We have had many conversations surrounding adoption, and feel this is something we would like to do after having our own biological children,'* says Nick. *'But when asked by someone who has their own biological children "why don't you adopt?" we think it is fair to bounce that question right back.'*

After much research, they have chosen 'gestational surrogacy' which will involve their sperm, a donated egg and a surrogate into whose womb the fertilised embryo is implanted. A close friend has offered to be an egg donor, but they have chosen to look to the US for a clinic and a surrogate. This decision was not simply based on what they felt was best for them; first, they worked through the wider implications of different options. *'We believe in ethical and legitimate surrogacy,'* explains Rory. *'We don't consider anything else a valid basis under which to bring new lives into this world. We are not prepared to exploit surrogates and legal loopholes in developing nations. We also want to avoid the uncertainties that changing political landscapes in some developing nations throw up. The favourable legal climate in the US means that all concerned are protected, and appropriately compensated for their part in the process.'*

Making it clear

Richard and his partner, Steven, are a British-American couple based in the UK. They also decided to find a surrogate through the US system. They believe that, with the right information, intended parents can manage the process, from choosing the surrogacy agency to choosing how many babies they will have. At first they struggled with the lack of clear and transparent information available. *'There was no information online and very few people had gone through this at that time,'* says Richard of his experience. '*So we just fell into working with an agency. We relied on the agency to tell us what was going to happen next, but they said they would tell us only when we needed to know. We soon learnt that even paying a lot of money doesn't always mean that you will receive the best service.*' This motivated Richard, once their children were born, to become an advocate, providing impartial advice and information, for other people (gay and straight) considering surrogacy in the US.

Luckily, Richard and Steven had friends whose twins had been born five years earlier, also via surrogacy in the US. This gave them some understanding of what was possible, despite many changes to the process even in that short time. It also meant they started with a clear idea of what they wanted. '*If you have a picture of the way you want your family, like we did, then you can align yourself with others who can help,*' says Richard. '*In the US, the IVF process is not like here, for some reason success rates are much higher. When we went through the process, it was aimed at enabling families to have twins. Two embryos from different sperm sources could be implanted into one womb, so both gay dads can each have a genetic link to one of the twins.*'

In the US system, most intended parents rely on their surrogacy agency to select a potential surrogate, rather than meeting surrogates informally first. '*The surrogacy agency has pages of information on you, they interview you and do a psychological screening,*' Richard explains. '*They are pretty quick at figuring you out and good at finding a match. First, we had a three-way Skype call – us as the intended parents, the surrogate and the agency. There was that initial awkward conversation, "so why do you want to carry our baby?" But if the agency's done their work properly, it should work.*' And, in this case, it did. '*I remember, after two minutes of talking to Angela, thinking, I love this woman, and she felt the same. We used up all of our air miles to fly over to the States five times during her pregnancy. We were lucky enough to be there for all of the scans, and of course the birth.*'

Richard, Steven and Angela remain in contact. '*She is still the most fantastic woman,*' says Richard. '*We send her photographs of the children and Christmas cards, as well as being friends on Facebook. She is and always will be a part of our family. Without her, our dream would never have become a reality.*'

Five things you should know

1. **There are different kinds of surrogacy.** The big distinction is between gestational surrogacy and 'straight' or genetic surrogacy. Both involve a surrogate: a woman who becomes pregnant and bears a child for someone else. In gestational surrogacy, the egg is donated by someone other than the surrogate. In genetic surrogacy, the surrogate's own eggs are used, so she and the child she carries will have a genetic connection, and insemination can happen at home or at a clinic. A gay male couple will usually use their own sperm to fertilise the egg.

2. **Surrogacy is legal in the UK as long as it's not commercial.** It's illegal for a third party (like a surrogacy agency) to provide matching services for profit, and you can't pay a surrogate or an agency more than 'reasonable expenses'. There are several agencies who can help – including Surrogacy UK, Brilliant Beginnings and COTS (Childlessness Overcome Through Surrogacy).

3. **Surrogacy can be very expensive.** If you are considering surrogacy in the US, then the legal fees, costs of IVF, fertility tests and other healthcare, your surrogate's expenses, air travel and time away from home and off work mean you could be talking about a six figure sum.

4. **You may have an ongoing relationship with the surrogate.** Before embarking on the process, contributors to this chapter did not anticipate that they would form a relationship with the surrogate herself, and often her family as well. While this does not happen with every family created through surrogacy, it can be an unexpectedly significant and enriching relationship.

5. **The law around surrogacy is complex and changing.** So get clued up, do your research and talk to people who have already become parents through surrogacy. Under UK law, the woman who gives birth is always treated as the legal mother and her husband or civil partner is treated as the legal father/other parent, irrespective of who the biological parents are. This means that, if you conceive your child through a surrogacy arrangement, you will need to obtain a parental order to reassign parenthood to you.

(*Source*: Brilliant Beginnings)

5

CO-PARENTING AND KNOWN DONORS

Known donor or co-parenting arrangements can be created between friends, acquaintances or people who have got to know each other simply in order to start a family. This way, the child will know who both their biological parents are and could have three or four parent figures in their lives. Each arrangement is different, so in this chapter we hear from a range of co-parents, parents, donors and donor-dads (sperm donors who understand themselves and are understood as the child's father) about how they chose this route; and what parenting means for them.

A way to make connections

Tricia and her partner's desire for a known donor came from '*a love of complex community and connection. We lived communally, believed it takes a village to raise a child and wanted to avoid nuclear family set-ups, so what's one more person added to the mix?*' So they put word out to friends and family that they were looking for a donor. Tricia's partner is Latin American, and they wanted to find a donor from her country. No luck. Then they looked on co-parenting and donor-matching sites. '*Just a depressing number of men looking to have sex, peppered with a few decent men who didn't request money or intercourse,*' says Tricia. '*We didn't end up contacting anyone.*' Next they took a more direct approach.

'*We asked two friends, both based abroad. We were such DIY feminist queers that we didn't fully appreciate that it helps to be in the same continent as the guy to get pregnant. Both completely ignored the question. Finally we decided to ask another gay friend of ours who we had discounted at first because his partner was so anti-baby. We emailed him to float the idea and got a warm response. He lived nearby and was older, which may have affected his readiness to consider the implications of being a known donor. He is the known dad, and plays a role like a special uncle, and his partner (a political, rabble-rousing artist and activist) is "naughty uncle".*

While her partner was pregnant, Tricia had doubts and worries, as well as joy and excitement, about the off-beat family they were creating together. *'As the non-bio mum I vacillated between fear that I'd be usurped as a parent and whole-hearted joy that someone might love our baby in some way that could match my partner's and my love for this kid.'*

A way to share the love

Lesbian mum Jessica and her partner wanted a known donor so that their children would know their biological father and *'there'd be no fantasy figure who was the best – or worst – person in the world'.* None of their friends seemed an obvious candidate, so they looked online. *'We knew we needed the sperm and wanted the friendship with the donor, but we did not want him to be involved in decision-making.'* But they struggled to find someone they clicked with.

A few months later, on a visit to university friends, over a late-night glass of wine, the conversation turned to their efforts to start a family. *'Our friend Simon said, "You know, I'd have done it if you'd asked me." And we thought, Why not? Simon felt it was a way to contribute. He didn't want or expect a parenting role,'* she says. *'He told us he would never have done this if he didn't think we'd be good parents. We had no in-depth discussions and no contract, maybe because we already knew each other so well, or because there was so little difference of opinion.'*

Lesbian couple Yasmin and Lizzie also felt strongly that they wanted their children to have a relationship with their fathers. They decided that having involved male parents in their children's lives was worth any extra complications that might bring. *'It was something we agreed on instinctively, without having to discuss it in detail,'* explains Yasmin. *'We both thought it would be important for our child not just to know who their father was, but to have a real relationship with him. We were lucky to be friends with a gay male couple who felt the same way, and we'd always joked about having children together. After lots of discussion, and a few wobbles along the way, the jokes became serious, and we decided to form a family together. Parenting with them has meant our daughter spends time with both sets of parents and has two mums, two dads and loads of adults who love her.'*

A way to keep control

Sally's daughter was conceived with sperm from a donor who she found through a matching website. She admits that at first she found it odd and uncomfortable to *'get in touch with a stranger and ask him for sperm'.* She changed her mind after speaking to a friend who had done just that. *'My friend pointed out that it wasn't that different from using a clinic, but cheaper and less exact,'* explains Sally. *'My partner and I would have full control over the choice of donor, and as civil partners we'd have legal rights as parents. So we set about looking for a donor online.'*

Meeting the donor, and choosing him themselves, meant that Sally and her partner felt better informed than they would have done choosing from donor profiles provided by a sperm bank. It also meant that they could inseminate at home, instead of in the medicalised surroundings of a clinic. They could tell their daughter as she grew older about the kind man who had helped them become parents, because they had actually met him for themselves.

However, first they had to meet someone. *'There were definite similarities to online dating,'* says Sally. *'When we found someone we thought we liked, we exchanged photos and arranged to meet in a café. Somewhere safe and public, as much for his benefit as ours. There we sat, teapot full, expectations high, and in he sauntered. He was in a relationship but didn't want children. He did, however, see the challenges some people face who do want them, and enjoys helping them. He didn't want a formal role in the child's life, which was fine with us. We had a lovely chat and resolved, by the end of it, that he could be our sperm donor.*

'The first time he came over to our home to make his donation, we ran round tidying up and anxiously tried to work out where he would like to provide his sample. When he arrived, we talked nervously, gave him the plastic container and watched him

disappear down the hall. The door shut and there was silence. In fact, there was far too much silence. What if we heard him "donating"! I immediately put on a CD and my partner went to empty the dishwasher.

'*After 15 minutes, he emerged, having left the sample on the bedside cabinet. I offered him tea and a biscuit – I felt it was only right. That's what they do when you give blood, right? He declined the offer politely and went on his way, wishing us luck. For many reasons it was impractical to stay in touch, but in another life I can see how we could have been friends.*'

It's a way to know the full story

While Sally, her partner and their donor were clear from the start that he would not have an ongoing relationship with them or their child, Sophie and her partner deliberately looked for someone with whom they could form a lifelong co-parenting relationship.

'*I was adopted as a baby and never felt like my adoptive parents were my true parents,*' Sophie explains. '*They were kind, loving, and gave me an excellent start in life, but I always felt a strong need to know where and who I came from. Aged four, I decided to find my biological parents, and 18 years later, I did. Every child is different – my adoptive brother has always seen our adoptive parents as his only parents. However, the emotional impact I experienced due to being adopted affected my decisions about parenting. I instantly ruled out adoption because I couldn't run the risk of a child struggling the way I did.*'

Sophie and her partner's first step was to build a profile on a co-parenting website. '*It was a bit of a minefield, especially as people become very particular when choosing someone to have a child with,*' admits Sophie. '*In a relationship you love someone so you don't mind that they have flaws, but in this situation suddenly people expect perfection.*'

Nonetheless, they found a guy they got on with and, after a few months of meeting up and getting to know one another, they started trying for a baby. He stopped being a stranger and became a friend. He soon became their baby's father. '*My partner and I are the predominant parents,*' explains Sophie. '*But our child and her father know each other and will develop a bond. We're considering drawing up a contract, so that we all remain on the same page no matter what happens down the line, but we haven't done so yet.'*

Tricia also advocates having a contract, even if you think you already agree on everything. *'It's not legally binding at all, but it is so worth going over issues, concerns and hopes. However awkward it might feel.* Especially *if it feels awkward,'* she urges, remembering the misunderstandings that arose between her and her partner and potential donors. *'This all needs to be clear and agreed beforehand or pain is likely to ensue when the tiny human arrives and there are different expectations. We downloaded a template off the Internet, changed it and used it to help discuss expectations.'*

Friendship, fulfilment and fear: What it can mean to be a known donor

What's it like to be on the other end of that email, call or conversation? To consider creating a new life, a child who shares your genes, but not be a primary or legal parent of that child? A man who donates sperm to a sperm bank will likely only ever know his biological children after they reach 18, if at all. However, a known donor is likely to see his biological children as they grow up and to be involved to some extent in their lives. It's an act of generosity which will have repercussions on his own life, as it did for James, Paul and David.

James had little idea what he was letting himself in for when his friends – a married heterosexual couple who were unable to conceive together – asked whether he would donate sperm in order to help them have children of their own. *'It happened a quarter-century ago in Los Angeles,'* he explains. *'I was living there for a year after university in the UK. Many people think of California as an incubator (no pun intended) for lots of social trends. Certainly in many parts of that state now, kids with two mums, two dads, or three or four parents don't raise eyebrows. But in the early 1990s it wasn't at all common.'*

James was in his early twenties at the time and barely knew any other LGBT parents. *'I had hundreds of gay acquaintances and friends,'* he says. *'But the only ones with children were those who'd previously been married to women.'* Having children would not have crossed his mind if his friends hadn't suggested it. For them too, this was a leap into the unknown. *'For a straight couple, like my friends, to have children through donor insemination was not so unusual. Having them with a donor known to you was considerably less common. Having them with your gay housemate was the kind of thing that could get you featured on a talk show.'*

His two daughters are now both young women, and James is satisfied with the role he has played and continues to play in their lives. It's a role that he and his friends worked out as they went along, with no models to follow. When the girls were young, James lived with the family, helping to look after his daughters each day. *'I changed nappies, prepared bottles and gave baths,'* reflects James. *'But I'd be the first to say that my friends were always the girls' mum and dad and shouldered nearly all the parenting responsibilities, both practical and financial.'* As they grew older and his own circumstances changed, he moved away and now has a less involved, but still emotionally close, relationship.

Over in the UK, at about the same time, Paul was considering a similar request: a lesbian friend had asked him to donate sperm so that she could have a child. At first, his feelings were mixed. He remembers, *'I had some pride in being asked, some nervousness about the implications and a sense that it was a good thing to do. The decision was pretty easy to make: I was an LGBT ally; this was a profound way I could do something positively life-changing for a good lesbian friend and there was no expectation of responsibility beyond delivering the first "act". It didn't feel like it would be particularly life-changing for me at the time.'* But Paul still had questions and concerns. *'There was a lot in the media about the new Child Support Agency (CSA) and attempts to get finances from "absent fathers",'* he says. *'I sought – and got – confirmation from my friend that she would not resort to the CSA in the future, although I didn't feel a need to get this in a legal form.'*

Paul and his friend Jackie agreed that he would not be expected to have contact with the child, so he didn't discuss becoming a donor with his family, only with a few close friends. *'I did not want to have to deal with others' expectations, issues, or prejudices,'* he explains. *'Looking back, it seems quite a clinical, uncomplicated way to take a decision to become a donor. And that reflects what was true at the time. There seemed to be very little information around: the Internet was in its infancy; national politics around LGBT issues were predominantly negative, characterised by Section 28, unequal ages of consent, no right to civil partnership or marriage; and gender parenting politics typified by issues like the CSA. The whole notion of what constitutes "family" is much more inclusive now.'*

It was a friendship made long before he ever considered being a parent that started David on the road to becoming a known donor. *'When I was 22, working in a restaurant, I made friends with a colleague called Antony,'* David explains. *'Twelve years later, when I bumped into him again, he was suffering from AIDS. In the months before he died I helped look after him, got to know his family and met his cousin Rosie for the first time. I didn't see her again for another eight years or so, and then her partner was heavily pregnant. They explained that the relationship with their donor was proving difficult and I said, "Well, next time, why don't you ask me?"'*

A couple of years later, when Rosie took him up on his offer, David had totally forgotten about their conversation. He didn't rush to respond, letting the idea settle, but soon realised that he really wanted to do this and wouldn't have the chance again. So he said yes. After that, it all moved quickly. *'We did have conversations before the birth, but not a great many,'* David recalls. *'Their stipulations were that there'd be no contact, just birthday and Christmas presents. Then if the child wanted to get in contact when they were older, they could. I thought, I'll deal with that when it comes, I'll just go with it now.*

'They sent me a kit with a syringe, and stayed in a hotel nearby for the weekend. I produced on the Friday and whizzed round with it on my scooter. They phoned the next day and said, "Can we do it again this morning, just so we have a better chance?" I produced again, handed over the semen and let them get on with it.' It worked! Rosie's partner was pregnant. David's job, it seemed, was done. They did not see each other again until after the baby was born.

'I asked to see them during the pregnancy because it all

seemed a bit surreal, but we never got round to it. I kept a low profile and thought, whatever happens, happens. I was able to compartmentalise it somehow,' he says. *'I didn't talk to anyone about it in depth. I told my best friend who said, "You must be mad." He was worried that there would be financial complications. It's such an off-the-wall thing to do, but at the time it didn't seem particularly crazy. I saw it as continuity in friendship, because of my relationship years before with Antony.'* Once the baby was born, David's role gradually changed. More than a decade later, he's now part of the family and sees his daughter every few weeks. However, things do not always work out so smoothly. *'I met a guy in exactly the same position as me,'* continues David. *'But it had been a very rocky road for him. He didn't get on with the mother. Eventually he decided to sever contact.'*

As a known donor, you might spend regular time with your biological children; you might just send Christmas or birthday cards; or you might not have contact until they are older. You are unlikely to have any role in decision-making or financial responsibility for your biological children, but you may develop a relationship with them. In a co-parenting arrangement, although the child or children may live most of the time with one set of parents, decision-making responsibility, and sometimes financial responsibility, is shared between all the parents. Co-parenting arrangements are more unusual. It can be hard to make them work: it can be tricky enough for two parents to agree on something, let alone three or four. Co-parenting can be disastrous if it goes wrong. Perhaps this is why it was difficult to find co-parents, particularly non-primary parents, willing to contribute to *Pride and Joy*. A child can legally only have two parents; other parents have few legal rights and can lose touch with their children if the relationship with the legal parents breaks down. But when it works, it means that there are more adults to love and care for the children, and a child can get to know all of their biological parents.

Five things you should know

1. **Know your rights (or lack of them).** If a lesbian couple in a civil partnership conceive with donor sperm, both mothers' names can go on their child's birth certificate.

This gives them equal parental rights and responsibilities and suits families where donors or donor-dads want to be involved with their children's lives but don't want parental responsibility.

Until 2009, it was possible to share legal parental responsibility between three or four parents in a co-parenting arrangement. This is no longer possible. If a lesbian couple in a civil partnership conceive with sperm from a known donor or co-parent, the biological father has no legal rights or obligations, even if all parties agree that they want him to. Even if a lesbian couple are not in a civil partnership, the biological father's name cannot go on the birth certificate if the child has been conceived through artificial insemination. This protects a donor-dad financially, but can be a vulnerable position for him if he wants to maintain an ongoing relationship with the child.

2. **It's worth taking time to talk.** Terms like 'co-parenting' and 'known donor' mean different things to different people, so it's important to get expectations clear from the start. These can be written down in a parenting agreement. Overleaf you will find a list of ideas about what to include. It won't be legally binding, even if you decide to take advice from a lawyer, but it is a gesture of intent.

3. **Your safety matters.** At a fertility clinic, all donor sperm is screened to make sure it doesn't carry sexually transmitted diseases. If you are planning to be a known donor, you will need to get these checks done yourself at a sexual health clinic or via your GP. If you are using a known donor, it's important for the health of yourself and your baby to be confident that the donor has a clean bill of sexual health. If you meet online or through a third party, take time to get to know each other. If anything makes you feel uneasy – from the obvious, like requests to have sex, to the indefinable feeling that something is amiss – don't do it.

4. **You can maximise your chances.** In this route, the method of conception is generally home insemination, informally known as the turkey-baster method or DIY-AI. If you're trying to get pregnant, tracking your cycle using ovulation tests or charting your temperature with a kit from any

high street chemist can help you work out when is the most fertile time in your cycle to inseminate. If you are the donor, it also makes sense for you to check your fertility before starting insemination in case there are any issues that will make it difficult to conceive.

Once you've checked the sperm are swimming in the right direction and circled those magic dates on the calendar, you're ready. The donor will need to ejaculate into a clean, dry pot. Twenty minutes later the semen has become runny enough to be drawn up into a needleless syringe which the woman inserts in her vagina. Beyond that, how quickly it works, or whether it does at all, is down to luck and Mother Nature. And yes, this is *all a bit awkward* – certainly the first time.

5. **There's no set pattern.** Known donor and co-parenting families are created for many different reasons and, whatever the initial arrangement is, it can evolve over time. Parents' or donors' views and desires can change once a baby is born and as relationships between parents and children develop. The stories in this chapter show that it's not just LGBT people who start their families in this way. Known donors to lesbians can be straight men. Gay men can help straight couples struggling to conceive. A straight woman can build a family with gay male friends. What matters most is the quality of relationship and communication between the parties. The possibilities are endless. You can find out more in chapter 13 'Nuclear explosion'.

Co-parenting or known donor agreements

Many people who enter into co-parenting and known donor relationships find that having some in-depth conversations about what to expect, before the conception or birth, prevents misunderstandings later on. Notes on what's been agreed upon are useful, but these agreements need to be tested out, discussed and amended, rather than carved in stone. This is a lifetime relationship between real people, not a warranty on a washing machine.

Below, you'll find some questions from Stonewall, which we've adapted a little. You may not have answers to them all, but they will definitely trigger some interesting conversations.

Practicalities
- Where will the child's primary residence be?
- How much time will each parent spend with the child?
- Will you have more than one child together?
- How will you decide the child's name and surname?

Legal considerations
- Who will be the legal parents?
- Who will apply for parental responsibility and how will they do it?
- How will you protect the status of any co-parents who do not have legal responsibility (for example, through your wills)?

Financial responsibilities
- Who will pay for what and how will expenses be divided between co-parents during the pregnancy and throughout the child's life?

Parenting
- Who makes the rules?
- How will you make sure your child receives consistent parenting?
- Will your child be brought up in a faith?
- How will your extended families be involved in the child's life?
- How and where will your child be educated?
- Who will attend parents' evenings?

Changes
- What happens if one of the couples splits up?
- What happens if someone dies?
- What if one of the co-parents or co-parenting couples wants to move away?
- How will you all make sure you discuss problems, questions or changes to any agreements as they arise?

6

STRAIGHT RELATIONSHIPS

In previous decades, most lesbian, gay, bi or trans people who became parents did so within a straight relationship. This is still the case today for many families, where parents come out or transition after their children have been born. There are also bisexual parents whose children are conceived through heterosexual sex, but who identify their families as queer or LGBT. This chapter shares experiences from these families; and gives advice to others in similar situations.

There are many reasons why people, who later identify as LGBT, enter into straight relationships or marriage. Lynn knew from childhood that she was a lesbian, but fear of what her family would think and a desire to be like everyone else propelled her into marriage in her early twenties. '*My dad was emotionally abusive, so I felt it would be safer to go the "normal route"*,' she explains. '*I got married when I was 22, had my first daughter at 23 and two other children shortly after.*' It took another two decades for her to pluck up the courage to leave her marriage, and finally to come out.

The turning point was when she realised that, although her marriage had brought her three much-loved children, it could not bring her happiness. '*A friend of mine came out later in life. I saw her moving on and being so much happier, while I was desperately unhappy. I thought I can't keep on like this any longer,*' she recalls. '*Before I made the decision to leave the marriage, I was doing a course in person-centred counselling. There's so much work as part of that about being authentic to yourself.*'

Once separated from her husband, Lynn was free to further explore her lesbian identity. But she was still a parent, and was keenly aware of the impact her coming out could have on her children. She made sure they heard it from her first. '*When we started on the divorce, I talked to the children straightaway. The youngest was 15. All three have multiple disabilities, including Asperger's syndrome. They all took it fairly matter-of-factly. My middle daughter said she'd seen that I was obviously not happy and was just waiting for me to tell her we were getting divorced.*'

It wasn't always that easy though. There were times when Lynn had to compromise and chose to put her children's needs first, even when they conflicted with her own. '*My coming out did create a few problems for my daughter,*' she remembers. '*She was studying at the same university where I worked, and so a lot of her friends knew me. Her best friend was keen on the Salvation Army, and my daughter was concerned it would ruin their friendship if her friend knew I was a lesbian. I didn't want to go back in the closet, and be out in some parts of my life but not in others, but I did. This wasn't a change my children had chosen, so I had to take things carefully.*'

Others get married for different reasons: Miriam and her ex-husband got married for the very simple, positive reason that they really liked each other. '*We've been best friends since meeting at university,*' Miriam explains. But was the depth of their friendship, which still continues today, a strong enough basis for marriage? They both thought so at first, despite some early warning signs. '*We had a discussion early on about how neither of us was entirely straight, but we ignored that and bumbled along for a long time,*' recalls Miriam. '*We both realised that we didn't want to marry anyone else of the opposite sex, so we fell into marriage with each other. A year in, I discovered he was bi. He had had an experience with a man before we were married, but was in denial.*' They carried on 'bumbling on', but that didn't work for ever.

'*Eleven years after we got married I met a woman and that started a chain reaction,*' says Miriam. '*We had a five-year-old daughter by then. I had about two weeks of thinking I was bi, then I realised, no, I'm a lesbian. That's when I said to my husband, "I can't stay in this marriage".*' In some ways, Miriam and her ex-husband were always an LGBT family, even if they didn't initially identify as such, even to themselves. The difference now is they can both freely own and express their

LGBT identities. One thing hasn't changed: they still remain friends, ready to share the care and responsibility for their daughter as she grows up.

Like Miriam, Katharine married young and is now separated from her partner. Fear of being different and social expectation both played a role in her decision, but primarily, she got married because she hoped marriage would 'cure' her of wanting to transition from male to female. *'When I was 12, maybe earlier, I was aware I wanted to have children, but I didn't expect it ever to happen,'* she says now. *'If I had transitioned in my early twenties, when I wanted to, I probably wouldn't have had children. Instead, I had a breakdown and was on a psychiatric unit for a short while. Once out of hospital, I got involved in charismatic Christianity. I married a woman in the young adults' group, because that was what was expected. That's when I thought marriage would cure me.'*

However, being married did not change Katharine's feelings, she still wanted to transition from male to female. At 32, with two sons, she decided that she couldn't *'live for someone else anymore'*. She chose to come out when her sons were so young – three and six years old – because she thought that would make it easier for them. However, it still took a long time for the family to adjust. *'I underestimated the impact on them,'* she reflects, now that they are teenagers. *'Even though the youngest doesn't really remember me as his dad, my oldest has taken a long time to get over the loss.'*

Katharine and her wife stayed together for two more years, but eventually the relationship broke down. Two years after that, with Katharine's wife unable to cope with parenting their two sons, the children moved in with Katharine; now they still see their mum each week. *'My narrative is very unusual,'* Katharine admits. *'I know of only four or five other trans single parents in the country.'* She is all too aware there are other directions her story could have taken: *'I know transwomen who have lost contact with their children and who have been in very difficult positions: one whose children have been brainwashed into not wanting to see her, another who was prevented by court order from contacting her children other than by letterbox. I'm not sure if orders like that are still being made, but I imagine it still goes on.'*

Katharine hopes her experience shows that another way is possible. *'I'd say to someone who's trans with kids and is thinking of coming out, you don't have to succumb to the narrative of transition, divorce, move away, never see your children again,'* she advises. *'There will be massive challenges, but it is possible. An increasing number of couples do stay together, or divorce and maintain contact.'*

Just because one partner in an opposite-sex relationship comes out or transitions, it doesn't have to mean the end of the relationship. In fact, despite the difficulties they have faced, Justine's relationship with her wife, Julie, grew in strength as Justine transitioned from male to female. *'In my twenties, I met the love of my life, Julie. We got married and had three amazing children. Life was good, but I always had that nagging voice in the back of my head telling me I wasn't being true to myself or others,'* Justine explains. *'By the time I was 36, I felt I could no longer hide who I was. I kept having the same dream. Although I am not religious, I dreamt I had died and was standing in front of God who asked me how I thought my life had gone. Truthfully, the only answer I could give was that I'd wasted it by not being myself and lying to others.'*

So one evening, despite fears of being thrown out into the street, losing her job, her marriage and her children, Justine sat Julie down and tried to explain. *'To my surprise and through many weeks of tears, we decided we would get through this together, just like in our wedding vows: "to have and to hold from this day forward, for better for worse, for richer for poorer, in sickness and in health, to love and to cherish, till death us do part."'* And they have. Even if to family, friends and neighbours, things seem to have changed, the love and commitment that created their family in the first place still remains.

Being bi or pansexual means that you could just easily fall in love with, marry and start a family with someone of any gender. That's why bi parents can be found in both same-sex and opposite-sex partnerships. Rebecca knew from a young age that she wasn't straight, but coming out to herself took many more years. *'I was raised in a very oppressive, religious environment and it took me a while to admit to myself and others that I was bi,'* she explains. *'I slept with girls at uni, but it wasn't until I was in my twenties that I really figured it out. I could not have been more surprised to find myself making babies with a guy. I had always wanted kids but didn't expect to end up having them with a man. I had vaguely planned to do IVF on my own once I got to 30.'* So what changed? *'Like many bi women, the respective size of the pool of potential male/female partners (and the fact my coming out predated Internet dating) meant that my mister turned up in my life just as I was plucking up the courage to brave the gay scene. Twelve years on, he's still awesome and we have two hilarious daughters, aged three and seven.'*

Naomi *'went through the confusion of being a teenager who thought I should be lesbian or straight. It was not until my early twenties that I realised I didn't need to be either. I had phases of identifying each way, but was looking to build my life with a woman – when I ended up with someone who identifies as male. We started a family in much the same way as any straight couple would; having one of each of what you need does make the job of conceiving a child a lot simpler! In lots of ways, our relationship looks like a fairly ordinary straight relationship, but it isn't.'*

Rebecca and Naomi are both women happily married to the biological fathers of their children. To outsiders, they may look as if they are in straight relationships, but they still identify as LGBT parents. Neither of them decided to enter an opposite-sex relationship rather than a same-sex relationship because it made it easier to become a parent: they simply followed their hearts.

Naomi's partner, Mina/Andy is gender-fluid, switching modes between more male or more female dress and identification. Naomi's pregnancy meant that they had to face up to questions about how open an LGBT family they would become. *'When I first fell pregnant it was hard, it was a tough time to work out what Mina needed to do,'* explains Naomi. *'It came down to this question: "Do we keep everything a secret from the child and have him miss a big chunk of his parents' lives?" While I was experiencing my body being pregnant, Mina came out more publicly and socially.'* Their decision during the pregnancy, to become more open about their LGBT identity, proved to be beneficial for their relationship with each other as they moved towards becoming parents. *'For me, it's been brilliant because I've got my full partner now,' says Naomi. 'For a year or so before I got pregnant, Mina had been in "boy mode", and I'd felt cheated – missing my wife because I only had my husband. Having a partner who is neither male nor female but is both feels like the full package. I can't quite explain, but now I've got the person I'm supposed to have.'*

The parents who contributed to this chapter had different reasons for starting their families in a straight relationship. There's no standard pattern for starting out (sort of) straight. But there are features these parents have in common: a commitment to their children, through changing and challenging times, and an LGBT identity – whether long suppressed, newly discovered or always a proud part of their lives.

Five things you should know

1. **There's light at the end of the tunnel.** Coming out later in life as a relationship ends can be tough on all sides, but it may be better than you expect. It can even be liberating. As Katharine says, there are plenty of other narratives apart from 'break up, move away, never see your children again' and plenty of families that reach crisis point and still find their way through to happier times. Don't let anyone else write the script for your life.

2. **People will want to define you.** If you come out after having children in a straight relationship, people may wonder if you are 'really gay' now. If you are bi or pansexual and choose someone of the opposite gender to be your life partner, people may assume that it was 'just a phase' and now you're straight. You don't have to accept these definitions, and shouldn't feel that you can no longer claim an LGBT identity simply because you're in a relationship with someone of the opposite gender.

3. **Plenty of people are in the same situation.** Some lesbians coming out in later life have found that they share a common experience with other lesbians they meet after coming out; although some felt judged by women in the lesbian community for having had straight relationships. Even if you feel isolated, you are not alone. Many people have walked this path before you.

4. **Your children can be your best allies.** Many LGBT parents put off coming out because they worry about their children's reactions. Your children are likely to have noticed if you are unhappy or hiding something from them, and talking to them honestly and in an age-appropriate way can be the best thing you can do.

5. **It's okay to seek out support.** You can find out more about adjusting to change in chapter 14 'Everything changes' or about forming, or maintaining, an LGBT identity in chapter 15 'Staying gay'.

Special Feature: Trailblazers

While there are still unique challenges facing LGBT families in the UK and Ireland – we wouldn't have written this book otherwise – overall, our lives are easier and more recognised now than at any other point in history. A significant part of this recognition is thanks to the experiences and the visibility of those parents who brought up their children at times when it was much more difficult.

This special feature takes an in-depth look at what it was like being an LGBT parent in the 1970s, through the experiences of Alan and Gill.

Alan

Alan married June in the early 1970s and they had two sons, despite Alan having known since childhood he was gay. It took many years of struggle before he came out, but the marriage survived and even grew stronger as a result.

I realised I was different when I was about ten, but I didn't have a word for it. The kids at school knew it too and I got a good bashing for it. At 15, I first heard the word 'homosexual'. I realised I was what my parents would have referred to as 'one of them'. I was terrified someone would pick up I was queer. I thought I'd be whipped into the nearest psychiatric hospital. My faith came into play too; I understood the Church's position was that this was a terrible sin. I prayed about it a lot, but it didn't seem to make any difference.

I entered a 20-year period of denial, where I tried to be 'normal'. I met my wife, June, then our older son was born in 1972 and the younger one in 1975. When they were both very small, I had a nervous breakdown. I was petrified of going outside. If I noticed an attractive man on the Tube on the way to work, I would feel guilty all day. I wondered how someone who was married with two children could cope with this.

I came close to terminating my own life. At the station on the way home, I thought I was going to jump. At the last minute, I panicked and ran away, up the stairs from the platform. I collided with someone who asked, 'Are you all

73

right?' It turned out he was a Samaritan. He persuaded me to join the local Campaign for Homosexual Equality group, and I later became the chair of the group.

I couldn't go on as I was, so I decided to tell my wife. That was the most difficult thing I've ever done in my life. I had to steel myself before I told her because I knew this could end our marriage. The first thing she said was, 'It must be my fault. I wasn't as available to you as a wife and a woman because we have two young children.' That was difficult to hear. But we talked for many hours, over many nights, and said, 'We'll see how things turn out.' We were still married 39 years later when she died. She was my best friend.

Being gay and married was more common at the time than I first realised. Many were living a secret double life. I went to a meeting for married gay people, expecting there would be few people as stupid or dishonest, as I saw it, as me. There were 30-odd people there! I came across a few other married gay people bringing up children, but I didn't get to know them well.

I felt I should tell other people once June knew, so she would have someone to talk to, although I was more inclined to come out than she would have liked. It wasn't easy or comfortable, but it did a hell of a lot to strengthen the marriage. In 1976, I went on my first Gay Pride march. There were as many police as people marching. Many were arrested for 'breach of the peace'.

My older son was a highly perceptive child, which led to difficulties, incidents which are now funny but weren't then. Once, he was opening Christmas presents with all the family. There was one from a gay couple we were friends with. 'This is from Terry and Tony,' explained Peter to his great-aunt. 'They are two men who live together and love each other very much' – you can imagine the look on her face!

I had a workroom, where I kept gay-related books and magazines. It was supposed to be off limits to the kids. When my older son was about six, he went into my room and picked up a gay magazine. He came and said to me, 'Daddy, what's gay?' I did my best to explain. He said, 'So Uncle Terry and Uncle Tony are gay?' 'Yes.' 'And you are too?' 'Yes.' He was quite accepting when I told him, he just ran back upstairs to play with his Lego. It was unexpected, so what I said was unplanned. After that, we always had a rule about being very honest with the kids, at their level of understanding. That continued as they became adults.

My youngest was also fine with it, and still is fine. He's not like his brother, who would badger you until he got an answer to something. My youngest is a truthful sort of soul; he just comes out with things. He used to worry June and me in that sense, because we could see the potential difficulties it could cause with peers.

The main thing difficulty with the children was being open with them at home, but telling them they couldn't shout it from the rooftops. That's why I stopped being chair of our local gay group. Sometimes the meetings would be reported in the local paper and my wife said, 'You've got to be careful with the children, they'll cop it at school.'

When my mother found out I was gay, she told me, 'I don't approve of you, I don't approve of your lifestyle, I don't approve of your friends.' I told her that if she felt like that, then she could stay away. I suppose that was unkind, but I was younger and more militant then. She was fine with the children, but she probably thought they were in some terrible situation. I think the argument about the impact on children is just cover for people who can't cope with gay people themselves. When I hear people talk about 'the children', I see red. Children are very accepting, provided they are loved and cared for.

Now I'm a grandfather. The reaction of my sons' partners and their families to me being gay is fine, I think. I suppose because I was always fairly militant: this is me, take it or leave it. I don't believe in being apologetic about who you are, and people seem to have always taken it in their stride.

I feel I was born too soon. I should be glad – I am glad – the rights we have today were all the things we were working for, but we never imagined any of this would happen in our lifetimes. I could not perceive there were real alternatives, and if I did, I couldn't take them seriously, because they weren't going to happen. At 16 I had a terrible crush on this boy, he never knew. In my fantasy world we were living together, but it was pure fantasy. I never dared to think it could ever happen. Homosexuality was decriminalised in 1967, but the impact was very limited. As activists, we thought if only we could get gays in the military or get an equal age of consent, that would be an achievement. Marriage was not even considered.

I'm immensely grateful that people can live their lives as gay people more easily than I could, but my gratitude is tinged with envy. What I would have given to have had that. I have a good circle of gay friends and I am still doing my best for the cause, but I sometimes wonder about what I could have done differently, whether there were things I should have tried to make possible.

Gill

Gill, a lesbian-feminist academic and journalist, conceived her son via artificial insemination from an unknown donor and brought him up in a lesbian household.

I was 30 when I had my son; I turn 70 later this month. My three ex-partners all played some part in my son's first eight years; and all three are friends of mine – two remain actively involved in aunt-like, or godmother-like, relationships with my son. My current partner and I have lived together for 31 years.

I was aware from early childhood that I wanted a baby. I played often with dolls and my battered pram. I don't remember ever wanting a husband and didn't know until later where babies came from. I was born in 1945 in Australia and had no idea there were LGBT parents. I had two girlfriends before I even heard the word lesbian.

I buried my desire for a baby during my university days, and when I moved to England and started work. Through feminist campaigning, I found out about artificial insemination (AI). Immediately my longing for a baby surfaced like a fountain.

I had a good male friend who I'd met teaching, and who I seduced after a college event. I knew very quickly that I was pregnant. I lost that baby at 19 weeks, but the experience of sharing the pregnancy with the baby's father, made me resolve to go down the AI route, since I had no intention of ever living with him. To begin a child's life with the intention of depriving a willing parent and helpless child of their possible relationship filled me with guilt. The 70s was a time of passionate feminism, anti-monogamy and experimentation. I already had a waiting family for a child: myself and my two partners. I was influenced by memories of a traumatic relationship with my own father, who had been bullying and misogynistic – and by my ardent feminism, which promised new and better ways for women and men to relate to one another. In addition, at that time there were no contested custody cases in the UK where a lesbian mother had been able to keep her child(ren). I didn't want to run those risks.

When my son was born, we were three mums: all bottle feeding, nappy changing, getting up in the night, and so on. The system turned me into 'Mother' almost immediately: NHS visits, decisions about vaccinations, application for Supplementary Benefits, and so on. My partners were freelance musicians and work had to come first for them. I was the decision-maker about babysitting, cooking, shopping, and so on. I was researching for my DPhil and teaching freelance for my son's first five years, so I decided to offer free board to an older woman in exchange for 20 hours a week babysitting. She fell in love with the baby, and he with her, and she became his beloved Nan. Sadly she developed breast cancer and died when he was seven.

For a while I felt I was the 'dad' – off to work to earn money after my doctorate: first typing in an office, then selling insurance, then as a journalist at *Gay News*. I'd get home tired and Nan would have my son fed and bathed, ready for his bedtime story. I felt competitive sometimes, and felt she was more 'mum' than I was. The others in the household did stints of help and childminding. I asked a gay male friend to teach him how to pee standing up – it didn't take long!

With respect to the system (NHS, Social Security, etc.), I behaved as if I were simply a single mother. I told no one in officialdom that I was a lesbian. I was offered adoption services by the hospital, who assumed I must have 'made a mistake'. I worried about the 'caring' professionals and sought to avoid them as much as possible. I was lucky to have support from my household (partners, plus friends) and my father and sister. I presented as a single mother and was only out as a lesbian in feminist circles.

I saw not being out as a lesbian mum as the best way of protecting my son, since I knew no other lesbian mums (or gay dads). On the other hand, I never lied to my son, nor hid anything, nor pretended heterosexuality, at home. I always answered my son's questions honestly, when he asked them, at a level I felt he could understand. He presumably grew up in two realities and lived two – just as I had, and did. If I had done otherwise, I'd have risked losing custody. Left-wing workers in the 'caring professions' might have been radical about social issues, but officialdom was very heterosexually conservative when it came to children and family. The Thatcher government had introduced Section 28, so school was a particularly perilous place for any lesbian mother.

During my son's first 15 years or so, there was a huge ideological divide in second-wave feminism between political (radical) lesbians (theoretically opposed and emotionally hostile to child-bearing) and socialist feminists (mostly hetero). There were also problems about having crèches at meetings and conferences: some fought against having boy children present, others argued that men should mind children to free women to attend meetings, others wanted no men anywhere in sight.

On the other hand, the gay movement was indifferent to children and knew nothing about their needs. My editor at *Gay News*, though a friendly gay chap, told me he'd employed me *in spite of* my being a mother. Arranging for school holidays was always a nightmare – I struggled with competing demands of job versus time with my son. Help never came from gay or feminist quarters, but from ordinary hetero neighbours or non-politico friends.

Once he finished studying, my son entered commercial life, completed an MBA and became, progressively, a successful manager, senior manager and executive. I have sometimes teased him about how establishment he has become, given his upbringing by a delinquent mother. Buying his first house, on a mortgage, he took in a lodger. He related to me that, at the interview, she had asked whether he'd mind her having her girlfriend overnight sometimes. He laughed and replied, 'Let me tell you about my mother...'

Special Feature: Seeking Asylum

LGBT rights in the UK have improved in recent years. However, there are still more than 70 countries where homosexuality is illegal, and five where it is punishable by death. In many cultures, LGBT people embark on heterosexual marriages and start families because they see no alternative or because they are forced to do so.

LGBT people who are refugees and asylum seekers in the UK have a legitimate fear that they will face abuse, imprisonment or even death if they return home. Many have experienced violence already. They may be detained or deported, if they cannot 'prove' that they are LGBT during the asylum process. In some cases, the fact that they have children is used as evidence against their claim, because of assumptions that LGBT people cannot or do not become parents.

Ram is a gay man seeking asylum in the UK. He has always dreamed of becoming a father, but knows that if he were to have a child, he would be unable to tell his family back home in India.

I grew up in a very conservative society. I'm not from a metropolitan city but from a Tier 2 city, and I lived in an environment which was as strict as a military school. There was no chance to get any insight into love or relationships. Even in my family, there was no talk of romance. I didn't realise when I was growing up that there was such a thing as 'being gay'.

In 2010, I came to the UK to study. I wanted to see more of the world. I didn't have time to explore much about my sexuality; I was busy studying, living on my own for the first time, and had to maintain everything on my own. But I had that spark now and again, the same feeling I'd had from a young age, so I finally found my courage to look online, because I experienced a huge physical necessity.

It was a big day for me. I was petrified even to look at a website, even though no one was watching. I met someone online and, on the first day we went out together, I realised this is what I am. I felt liberated and very, very worried at the same time. I had been told all my childhood how an adult human being should be, and being gay was the opposite of all I'd been told.

I felt there was something wrong with me. A friend advised me to speak to a doctor. I thought he'd gone mad – how could I speak to the doctor about this? I wasn't out, only a couple of people knew. I was very frightened. I gathered up all the courage in my soul and went to the doctor. I was hesitant even to say the word 'gay'. Luckily it was not an Indian doctor, I couldn't have told them, the slightest reaction would tell me what they thought. I had lived in India for 25 years, I knew what people would think, even my family wouldn't have been able to accept me. The doctor referred me to an LGBT organisation and I met other gay people.

It was a roller-coaster ride of feelings. At one point, I felt fine, at another point, I knew this was totally different to how I had been brought up. Going to the wedding of a friend and his male partner changed my whole perception. Both families were there and a huge crowd. It was breathtaking. I felt such happiness. I was slowly realising that being gay, even being married, is fine here, and very, very normal.

I have always been passionate about having children. Around this time, I started finding out about how I could become a dad. I'd heard about test-tube babies, but I didn't know anything about surrogacy. I read all about surrogacy and realised that, even with being gay, I could still have my family. I emailed private clinics in India to find out if this was possible, but there was nothing for gay or lesbian people, or single people. That door closed for me. I realised significant stigma was attached, even for a single heterosexual person, let alone homosexual.

I started finding out about adoption. In India, people would say, 'It's not your child, why should you care?' But I see it as giving life to a child. You don't have to give birth in order to have a child. You can give birth from the heart. I went to the council office, but I still thought that you couldn't apply to be an adoptive parent if you were gay. Twice, I asked them 'Is it okay?' and when they told me I was eligible, I was very relieved. But I shared a house, and realised it would be better to have my own house before I applied to adopt. I was also applying for asylum, and everything in my life was upside-down. So I thought I need to wait until I am more stable myself.

Then one of my friends told me that he had registered at a co-parenting website. On the same night, I started looking into it. I thought I could be a co-parent or a donor. People I met through the site kept asking me whether I would donate sperm, but I wanted to be choosy. Creating a life is an auspicious thing; you don't just do it for fun.

I met a local lesbian couple through the site. We've been trying for a few months. We have a good rapport, a comfortableness together. We don't have an agreement, although we have talked about the child knowing me as the biological father when they are older. One of them got pregnant, but had an early miscarriage. I am praying for them. Even if I am just a donor, that would be lovely. I could still visit the child because of the friendship I have with this couple.

I go on dates, and some of the people I've met are not happy with the notion of having a child. I wouldn't want to enter into a relationship with someone like that. Being a parent is an absolute necessity for me, and I can feel it in my bones. For me, a relationship has to be for a lifetime. I was brought up with that idea. Once a marriage is done, it's for life.

I can't imagine gay and lesbian people being accepted in India in my lifetime. It's hard to make people understand what it is to be gay, let alone to accept it. If I did become a father, I don't think I'd be able to tell my mum, which is really sad for me. I'd be really excited to tell my mum, she's helped me such a lot and made such sacrifices for me, but I couldn't tell her, because she would be unable to accept me as gay. For some reason, I think she knowingly ignores and wants me to get married to a girl, though we haven't spoken about it openly, as it's taboo to speak about romance and sex.

I'm in the process of seeking asylum. I've read about atrocities carried out on the LGBT community in India, where people kill their own children to preserve the family status. It's really opened my eyes. India can be a hell for gay people. I don't think it's okay to send people back; it's really not okay. You might think people would concoct lies about being gay to stay in this country, but I tell you, people might lie about other things, but no one would lie about being gay because of the social shame of being thought to be gay, in countries like India.

They say, in a big city like Mumbai, it's okay to be gay. But that's not my home; I don't even speak the language. Being gay is still illegal there, people can beat and kill you. Even if you've lived somewhere a long time, you are not safe. If you come to a new place and they find out you're gay, there is twice the risk. You need a sixth sense to know if someone is okay to trust. Nobody can live a life like that, with threats or in the shadows.

I don't know anyone here who has been successful in an asylum claim. I read online about an Indian couple who were in a closeted relationship, who were told it will be okay if you go home. As long as you don't tell anyone, you will be safe. But that's not the case with me, as I am already completely out. I cannot create a family anywhere in India. I want to make my life here, this is my home.

Part Two

Coming out as a family

7

THE NAME GAME

This chapter explores the significance of naming; uncovers some of the different names that LGBT parents choose for themselves; and shares tips about choosing names.

Names arouse strong feelings. Most parents spend hours, days, even months, discussing names for their child. For LGBT parents, as well as resolving what you're going to call your children, you have to decide what they will call you. When a parent transitions, when children get older or when a new partner joins the family, new names may develop and old ones may be left behind.

Follow tradition
Well, as traditional as it gets for alternative families. 'Mummy and Mama' or 'Daddy and Papa' tend to be popular names for same-sex parents. 'Mummy' takes no explaining: everyone knows what a 'mummy' is. A 'mama' is more of an unknown quantity, but is becoming a name that many proudly claim. Adoptive parent of two Carla is one of them. *'At first, we were going for "mum" and "mummy"',* she says. *'But we realised it was unlikely that any child was going to say "mummy" for the rest of their life. So now we are "mummy" and "mama". It's great being a mama, even though you can never get cards with "mama" on in the shops.'*
   Many people assume that 'mummy' designates the birth parent or main carer. While for some couples it does, others, like lesbian parents Marie and Beth, choose to turn this assumption on its head. Acknowledging their concern that Beth, as the non-birth mother, would not be seen as a 'real' mother, they decided that Beth would be 'mummy' with all

the legitimacy and recognition which that name brings. *'I had the genes, so our son got Beth's surname and Beth got to be "mummy" while I am "mama",* says Marie. *'You wouldn't have thought it made much difference, but it helped Beth to feel more socially accepted as our son's mum. It's not bothered me. I'll always know that I carried him for nine months.'*

'My partner calls her mother "mam" so we felt it was natural she would be mama and I would be mummy,' explains Kim, who was the birth mother for their first child but not for their second. *'Our children have never questioned this, but adults find it very difficult. We often got asked how we decided who would be called what. We found it strange that, when my partner became pregnant with our second child, family and friends asked what this child would call us,'* recalls Kim. *'They seemed to insinuate that the term "mummy" should be for the biological mother only, and that we should be called different names by different children depending on who had given birth to them.'* Kim and her partner did not take up this idea. They were already mummy and mama. The idea of one of their children calling Kim 'mummy' and the other calling her 'mama', based on whether or not she was their birth mother, would be confusing and unnecessarily privilege the biological parent.

Make it fair

'Before our children were born, my partner said she wanted to be Mummy, so I said I'd be Mama,' explains Jenny. *'But as it got nearer, I thought, No, no, I want to be called Mummy. If they are in the park and call "Mummy", I want that to be me. So we decided to be "Mummy Jenny" and "Mummy Lucy". Now, they sometimes call us both "Mummy" and sometimes call us by our first names.'*

Scott and Tris started off as 'Daddy Scott' and 'Daddy Tris', but this only lasted a few weeks after their sons were placed with them for adoption. *'We then became "Dad" and "Daddy",'* says Scott. But now their sons are teenagers, this has changed again: *'It's "Dad" and "Dad" these days, but we all know to which dad they are referring by their tone. It's a very bold and matter-of-fact "Dad" for my partner, and a softer "Dad" for myself.'*

Be creative

If you don't feel comfortable with conventionally feminine names like 'mummy', 'mum' or 'mama', there are other options. Sophie says, *'I've always wanted to be a mum, so it was automatic for me to be "Mummy", especially as I carried the child and am the biological parent, but my partner is gender-fluid and has always felt more of a dad than a mum, so we wanted to incorporate that into the parental name. We spent ages working it out, but they are predominantly known as "Papa". We also use "Papa Bear" and "Mummy-Papa".*

'*We have come up against some opposition in using a male parental title for a female person. Some people feel that is confusing. But we feel this way is true to who we both are. Who you are as a parent is about who you are as a person, not a gender, and not a sexuality. As our child gets older we will explain all of this to her and she can choose what to call us.*'

Inspiration is all around. Sara explains, '*My partner didn't want to have a mother-type name. We tried and tried, but we still hadn't found a name by the time our son was born. Then we saw a trailer for some children's film – The Last Mimzy – so I am "Mummy" and she is "Mimzy". It caught on.*'

If two partners in a couple have different nationalities, native languages or backgrounds, they can choose parental names from their different cultures. This not only helps distinguish between the two dads or two mums, but also, in a small way, passes on an understanding of the family's heritage to the children. Lil is British but her partner is Japanese, and they have chosen names which reflect their different backgrounds. '*Japanese is convenient as there are two words for mother,*' explains Lil. '*My partner is "Okasan" which is the more traditional or formal word for "mother", and her older children already call her that. I am called "Mama", or in English, "Mummy".*'

Not everyone goes for this idea though. '*We went for "Daddy" and "Papa",*' says father of two Dónal with a tinge of regret. '*My partner is from Alabama, but refused to be known as "Pa" (pronounced "paw") like in The Waltons. I think he's depriving the boys but hey...*'

First names come first

Some families do away with 'mum', 'dad' or other traditional parental names altogether. There are many LGBT families where children call one or more of their parents by their first names, and just as many different reasons for doing so.

A generation ago, it was more common for first names to be used for non-biological parents, and still today, for new partners joining the family after the children are born. Bryony, brought up by her mum, her mum's female partner and her dad, says, *'I call my birth mother "Mum", because she is my mum and always has been. I call my father "Dad" for the same reason. I call my mum's partner by her first name as that's what she was introduced to me as when I was five. I also call her by her nickname and we have pet names.'* Jess, now in her twenties, also grew up calling her biological mother 'Mum' and her other mum by her first name. *'I think my parents implemented this to avoid confusion,'* she says. *'I suppose, also, there were very few other LGBT parents at the time and they didn't have examples to follow.'*

Known donors also lack examples to follow to help define their roles. They can fulfil a role which is fatherly, yet not a full-on, full-time dad. Some are happy to be known as 'dad', others prefer to use their first name, rather than a parental role name. This is the case for David, who donated sperm to lesbian couple Nicki and Rosie. He sees his daughter and her brother every few weeks, but he has no formal parental responsibility. *'They just call me David, not Dad,'* he explains. *'The children seem very happy with that. We've always told them the truth and it's never been an issue as far as I'm aware.'*

However, some families have found that the names their children use change depending on age and context. Jessica and her partner asked a friend to help them start their family. Like David, he's part of the children's family without having parental responsibility. It's a role that's clear within the family, but can be hard to explain outside it. Jessica explains how it works for them: *'The children are very open at school that they have two mums and a dad. They call him Simon, but they refer to him as "Dad" to other people. They are clear that my partner and I are their parents, but Simon is their dad.'*

Using her first name with her children also helps Katharine, who is a single parent who transitioned when her two sons were three and six years old, to be clear about her role. Now in their teens, they have called Katharine by her first name for as long as they can remember. Katharine prefers this because *'they've already got a mum and it was never my intention to try to be that role'*. She's no longer their dad, and doesn't want to replace their mum, so using her first name seems the best answer.

Let your children decide

If you put off the decision for long enough, this will happen anyway. Some parents find this difficult because you need names to refer to yourself and your partner from day one. It is a strange feature of early parenthood that you are so often referred to in the third person that you take to doing it yourself, like a member of the royal family. Adoptive parents need to decide how they refer to themselves, so the child can find out about them before they first meet, but these names are not always the ones which stick. *'You make a book before you meet them, pictures of the dog, the garden and so on,'* says adoptive mum Alison. *'We decided I would be called "Mummy" and my partner would be "Mum" and we put that in the book. But he started calling us "Mummy" and "Mumma", and uses "Mum" generically for both of us. He'll bellow "Mum" and we'll both say, "Yes darling."'*

Eight-year-old Adam has it all worked out. When asked what he calls his parents Jo and Heather, he quickly replies, *'Parents of doom!'* before explaining how it works in his household: *'I call Mummy, "Mummy", because she used to call her mum, "Mum", and I thought I would need to call my mummy something different. I thought if I called Mama "Mummy" too, then if I shouted up the stairs they wouldn't know who I was calling for. I used to mix up my mums' names and call them both "Mumia" – and they mix up my name with my brother's, or even the cat's.'* He only sometimes comes across an awkward situation *'When people think my mummy is my nan.'* Many LGBT parents will have come across such situations, where strangers try to make sense of their family in a more conventional way, rather than seeing the relationships in front of them (*'I'm not that much older than Jo!'* adds Heather).

Victoria's son is younger than Adam, but has already come up with his own names for his two mums. *'My partner is "Mum" and I am "Mumma" or "Mum-mum",* says Victoria. *'He figured a way to differentiate for himself. However, he has recently taken to calling me "Victoria Lawson", I think because he hears other people calling me that. I wonder if the neighbours think that's what we told him to do!'*

There's only one mum in Bronwen's family – and it's her. Bronwen adopted her daughter when she was nine and old enough to decide for herself what name – or names – she would use for single-mum Bronwen. *'I get called Mum, Mumsie, Mother, Mama, Mother dearie,'* lists Bronwen. *'I think my daughter likes to try out all the possibilities she can, now that she has a mum!'*

Susie also answers to different names, depending on the social context and her children's needs. She knows that her son and daughter are still getting used to her transition to female and need reassurance that the loving relationship hasn't changed. *'My oldest calls me "Susie", and occasionally "Mum" if we are out, and that helps other people to understand our relationship,'* explains Susie. *'My youngest alternates between "D", "Susie" and sometimes "Dad". When they're sad about something they are more likely to call me "Dad". They rarely "Dad" me in public though and they know there are some places where they must never do it, like when we're swimming or I'm in the queue for the ladies".*

It was simpler for Justine, who also transitioned when her children were growing up. *'I've been lucky. Right from the start, my kids have been happy to call me "Mummy" and my wife, Julie, "Mum",'* she says. Her older daughter, Samantha, explains how it happened: *'One night my brother, sister and I decided, we've now got two mums – we can't have "Mum 1" and "Mum 2". So we carried on calling mum "Mum", and started calling Justine "Mummy".*

What's in a name?

If you are a woman out with a child, people will assume that you're 'mummy' regardless of what you call yourself or your children call you. *'When the children are with my partner, who they call "mama", and people say things like, "Go to your mummy," the children look confused because they know Mummy isn't with them,'* says Kim. *'Our youngest has started to say, "That's not my mummy," which makes my partner look like she has stolen a child!'*

The assumptions other people make about her family have made Kim think again about her own use of language: *'It made me challenge myself about how I speak with children. I realised I would sometimes refer to mummies and daddies, now I generally refer to a parent or carer instead.'*

It's not just parental names that are carefully chosen, children's names are too. Birth parents rarely reveal their choice of names until their baby has arrived. At that point few people would dare say anything apart from 'how lovely' about the choice of name. However, with adopted children, people can be more inclined to pass judgement.

'His birth mum chose our son's name, and it is quite unusual,' says adoptive mum Alison. *'Before we met him we wondered about calling him a different name, but when we met him, we knew, yes, that name was definitely him. People say, "Ooh, that's unusual, have you thought of changing it?" and then, even when we say no, make suggestions of names we could call him instead.'*

It is respectful to parents and children if we listen to the names people give themselves, and use them correctly. Shoshana, who was raised by lesbian mums, says that *'every family has its own language'* and she's right. Decisions about naming are very personal. They may be different from the ones we make for ourselves, but they all deserve respect.

'Sometimes I'm dubious,' Shoshana admits. *'I used to babysit two children of a lesbian couple, who knew one member of the couple as their mummy, and the other by their first name (a naming structure which belied the family relationships). I'm not a fan of granting parents radically different positions in a family. However, I recognised that was how that particular family had chosen to relate to each other, so I respectfully repeated their language whenever appropriate.'*

Selecting surnames

Will the whole family take one parent's surname? Will you create a new name? Or, will you have different names within one family? It's another sensitive issue, influencing not only what your child is known as, but also how people see your family connections. It can mean passing on or giving up something precious to you: your family name and associated sense of identity.

This issue isn't unique to LGBT families. There are many straight women who keep their original names after marriage, at least in a work context, a few straight couples who combine their names or double-barrel, and fewer straight men who take their partner's name. Perhaps it is harder for straight families to break with tradition and buck the trend, whereas LGBT families have already ripped up the rule book and have the chance to rewrite it.

While double-barrelled surnames are becoming more common – a meet-up of LGBT families now sounds more like a gathering of the aristocracy – naming conventions struggle to cope with co-parenting, multiple-parent, separated or blended families.

When Rosie's children were born, she couldn't put her name on their birth certificates alongside her partner's. There was just a blank in the space for 'father's name'. But naming her children helped to stake her claim to parenthood. '*We gave them a combination of our surnames, so they could be symbolically part of me too,*' explains Rosie. But as the children have got older, they've expressed their preferences and naming has become a live issue again. '*My partner and I didn't change our names, but now our children want us to have the same name as them. I don't want to change my name. Even after we had our civil partnership, I wanted to keep my own name. It's my individuality.*' The debate continues.

Han was born in the early 1990s and her mums faced the same problem, but resolved it differently. '*I have my non-biological mother's last name,*' Han explains. '*I think that this is really important and has helped other people view her as my parent. It makes the whole thing more equal. I imagine it also made it easier for her side of the family to accept me as part of them.*'

Victoria's son was born more recently, at a time when, as the non-biological mother, she can take her place on the birth certificate too. So she's less bothered about whether or not her name lives on in his. '*I was going to change my surname, but in the end I was too lazy,*' she admits. '*He has my partner's surname, which is fine. A lot of our straight female friends have a different surname to their kids, if the child has the father's name, but they've kept their own name. It's one of the things people obsess about before the birth and that don't matter at all afterwards.*'

Top tips

1. **Think about the message you're sending.** Names are not just convenient labels. They have always been used to describe the significance of different family roles. So whether you want to stick with or mess with traditional names and naming conventions, be aware of the signals this sends out about who and what matters in your family. You can use names creatively to ensure that non-bio parents, co-parents and donor-parents are all valued and validated as part of the family.
2. **Don't limit yourself.** LGBT families don't have to fit into boxes. Because our families are only just being acknowledged publicly, we have the opportunity to question names and roles. You can create your own surname, use traditionally gendered names across genders, have two of the same name or abandon 'mum' or 'dad' altogether.
3. **Be flexible.** Names change over time. Daddy may become Dad. First names may replace parental names, or vice versa. Your relationships with your children grow and change, and the names you choose could do as well. They may also change depending on the context – your children may call you by your first name when you're together, but 'Dad' when they're talking to friends at school.
4. **Be comfortable.** You may need to try a few names for size before finding the right one. If it's something you're happy for your children to yell down the stairs or across the park at you, then you're on to a winner.

8

FAMILY VALUES

This chapter discusses telling your parents about your own parenting plans; suggests how to cope with family rejection; explores how to deal with questions from your family; and celebrates the joys of extended families.

It's shifting now, but there is still an assumption that if you identify as lesbian, gay, bisexual or trans, you're not going to be a parent. And if you're a parent, well, clearly you can't really be LGBT. Just by existing, LGBT parents show that this isn't the case. By living and loving in the families that we do, a whole bunch of people – our mums, dads, grandpas and grannies, cousins, siblings, in-laws, great-aunty Maureen and all – can get to know and become advocates for LGBT families. It's a position they might never have sought out, but which many now choose to embrace. Sadly, there are also families who choose differently, and who will not accept their children or build relationships with their grandchildren, nieces or nephews.

Telling your parents

It starts when you come out. There's a conversation with your parents, maybe tears, probably questions about whether you're really sure, and hopefully hugs and declarations of love and acceptance. Then they say it: 'We'll never be grandparents' or 'Don't you want to have children?' or 'But you'd make such a great dad/mum'.

Jackie came out as a lesbian in 1975, when she was 22. Her mother's first response was to urge her not to tell her father and her second was to hope that Jackie would meet a nice Jewish girl. *'The next thing she said to me was, "I'm not going* to become a grandmother,'" remembers Jackie. There was no doubt in her mother's voice. That was just a statement of fact, one which Jackie internalised for nearly 15 years, despite her desperate desire to have a child.

The visibility of LGBT parents and the legal protection for same-sex relationships has changed almost unrecognisably since the 1970s. Yet when Alison came out to her parents, more than 30 years after Jackie did to hers, she got a remarkably similar response. 'I'd just turned 25 when I came out,' explains Alison. 'I'd been in a relationship with a male partner for six years. My mum's first reaction when I came out was: "How can you be gay, I thought you wanted children?" To her, a relationship meant being able to have babies in the "natural" way.'

When he was growing up, Scott had assumed that because he was gay, he would never be a parent. He gradually overcame his doubts and fears about being a gay father, and he and his partner applied to adopt, but he still had to tell his parents about his plans. Years before, it had taken him a long time to pluck up the courage to come out to them, and their reaction had been mixed. 'My mum told me to be careful and safe, and if I ever needed to, to talk to someone I could trust,' he says. 'My dad was another story, unfortunately we did not speak for a few months and, when eventually we did, it was very difficult. I expected a similar reaction to our plans to adopt. Surprisingly, this time, their reaction was excellent. Of course, they had their doubts, we all did, but they were very keen on us adopting.'

If your family struggled when you came out, it's natural to worry that it will be just as uncomfortable telling them that you're going to become a parent. But this is not necessarily the case. Your parents might not have known any other LGBT people before you came out to them. They may have had alarming assumptions about what life is like for LGBT people, based on what they've seen in the media or heard when they were growing up. But they do know what it's like to be a parent. Announcing your plans for parenthood is different from coming out: you are rejoining the mainstream, rather than setting yourself apart as a member of a minority group.

When Felix came out to his parents, they took a little while to get used to the idea. 'When I first told my mum, she burst *into tears and said, "You'll never have a child,"* he recalls. But the family is now '*100% positive. If my dad had not had a gay son he'd not be particularly pro, but now he couldn't be more so. Coming out was hard. Telling them they'll get grandchildren, well, what more could they want?*'

But what about if you come out when you've *already* got children? People often assume that you can't *really* be LGBT because you're a parent. You must be mistaken. It must be a phase... All the anxiety of coming out for the first time might then also be exacerbated by dealing with separation, divorce, custody arrangements or adjusting to being a single parent at the same time.

Poppy, who has one young son, came out as bi when she was a GCSE student at a girls' grammar school. She didn't publicly identify as lesbian or look for a same-sex relationship until after her son was born. Her teenage years were a confusing time, and having support from her parents was hugely important. She explains, '*The school was very proper. People didn't think that being gay was socially acceptable. I came out as bi rather than lesbian to soften the blow. Everyone was fine to my face, but some girls were bitchy behind my back. Whatever happened at school, I was always accepted at home.*'

Being out as a teenager wasn't easy. '*I didn't know any LGBT people. I was confused by how different I felt to other girls,*' she says. '*So I carried on dating guys. I felt pressurised into having sex. Not that anyone said you must do it, but I was a virgin and I'd come out as bi, how much more could I stick out? I had just turned 16 when I found out I was pregnant.*'

Poppy's parents have always been there for her, but that doesn't mean that, even now, they totally understand her identity and experiences. '*People do ask me, "How can you have a child if you're gay?"*' continues Poppy. '*Lots of people can't get their heads around it, even my girlfriend's family, even my mum, but if no one tries to explain, no one will ever understand. It's lack of education and fear that leads to homophobia. I want people to learn from my experience.*'

Unlike Poppy, Susie had left home and started her own family long before she came out to her parents. Her parents are divorced, living on opposite sides of the globe, but they have both supported her throughout her transition from male to female. '*My mum is fine about it, she's very invested in what I'm doing without being stifling,*' says Susie. '*My father is in Australia, I've not seen him for years, although we talk on the phone. It helps my children that both their grandma and their grandpa are fine with it.*' Knowing that her parents still love and support her in her new identity has enabled Susie to ask them to do something very special for her. She explains, '*I said to my mum and dad, "You named me when I was born, will you help choose my name now?" They did, and coincidently they both chose the same name.*'

Deciding when to tell

If you are already out as LGBT and planning to have children, when is the right time to tell your relatives? No different to anyone starting a family, this a personal decision which depends on the kind of relationship you have, how much you might look to them for support – and how long you think they'll need to get over the shock.

Peter and his partner are at the very start of the adoption process. They have spent hours discussing their hopes and fears with each other and contemplating what parenthood will be like. As they felt confident of a positive response from their families, they wanted to include them in these discussions, even if it will be months before a child is placed with them.

'*Some people might consider sharing this information so early on as a mistake, or something that should be avoided to prevent a barrage of questions and pressure, but that wasn't an issue for us,*' reflects Peter. '*My mum asked how, where and when, saying, "I never thought you would want to be a parent." She is excited about having another grandchild. My partner's mum, who already has seven grandchildren, also loved the idea. I pictured her planning a reshoot of the grandchildren photo with a space for our little gem.*'

For some, like Peter and his partner, sharing the ups and downs of their journey to parenthood with their families can be a source of support. For others, it can add to the pressure of an already stressful situation. '*We didn't tell our families for a long time that we were trying to get pregnant,*' says Victoria, a non-bio mum whose son is now three years old.

While they were open with friends and with Victoria's employer, who enabled her to take the time off that she needed for appointments, they held back the news from their families. *'Our families are completely fine with us being gay,'* affirms Victoria. *'But we didn't want to talk about trying for children with them. It was such a long and painful process, we wanted to forget about it and talk about something else when we saw them. In hindsight, I would have told them earlier. The first my partner's mum knew was when I phoned her from the emergency ward to tell her that her daughter was having an ectopic pregnancy.'*

David also left it until the last minute – until after his daughter was born – before telling his family. Despite a good relationship with them, he was unsure about telling his parents that he had donated sperm to a lesbian couple. The agreement was that he would only have limited contact with the child, so he worried whether it was really right to involve them if they wouldn't know this child as part of their family. Would the news shock or upset them too much?

'I told my sister, seven months into the pregnancy,' David explains. *'She said, "You must tell Mum," but I said no. Recently, my mum had been diagnosed with a terminal illness. A couple of months after that, my dad had dropped dead in front of her. She'd had these major shocks. I didn't want to tell her in case anything happened, like a miscarriage or a problem at the birth, in case she thought she was jinxed.*

'So I waited until the baby was born. When I told her, she said disbelievingly, "Well, I don't know, the things you get up to," and I thought, That was easy. But half an hour later she started crying and cried for hours. She cried because she didn't have my dad to tell and he would never know his grandchild. After the birth, I saw the baby every six weeks or so and her mothers enabled her to meet her grandma, my mum. She was thrilled. I felt that I was giving my mum something she never expected to have from me – grandchildren. She died a year later.'

Helping your family to adjust

When you announce that you're thinking of becoming parents,

not all family members will pop open the champagne. Some might be over the moon, especially if they've always known you wanted children, but many will be surprised and unsure at first. That doesn't necessarily mean they aren't supportive, but they may have worries which are hard to talk about – ranging from what their friends will think, to the impact on the child of having LGBT parents, to the ethics of assisted conception. It may take them weeks, months or even years to get used to the idea, especially when it is just an idea. The turning point often comes when it stops being an idea, and becomes a child.

'*My family struggled with my way of having a child*,' explains Chantelle, who conceived her daughter with help from a friend who donated sperm. '*Adoption would have made more sense to them, but they didn't get this. They liked my partner and thought she was good for me. But me getting pregnant in the way that I did was a step too far. We'd got married with both of us in white, with all my Cypriot relatives watching, and now they had to support me having a baby with someone they don't even know. But as soon as my daughter was born, no one asked, no one questioned, no one cared. She is so close to my family, they adore her. There couldn't be a more perfect bond.*'

Lea, who's pansexual, found that while her parents were initially unsure about her decision to start a family, due to her visual impairment, physical health and history of mental health, they too are now smitten with their granddaughter. When she started planning to have a child, Lea was married to a transman and explored getting donor sperm on the NHS. After a long wait and little success, she approached a friend to be a known donor. She got pregnant first time. Like Chantelle's parents, Lea's mum was already used to a few surprises from her daughter, even before her phone beeped one day at work. '*I told my mum by text that I was pregnant and then we texted back and forth*,' remembers Lea. '*Her first question was, "How? He lacks the equipment!"*'

Having told her mum – and survived – Lea was reluctant to tell her dad. She explains why: '*He reads the* Daily Mail. *He never smiles. He's known to all who know him as Mr Grumpy.*' And yet once his granddaughter was born, he changed. '*Now all he does is smile when he's with her*,' beams Lea. '*A colleague of his said to me, "Why didn't you have a child earlier? Your dad's got a sense of humour now!"*

While the reality of a grandchild plays a huge role in melting hearts and changing long-held views, so does the influence of other family members. Nicki found this out when she got pregnant with help from a known donor. '*My mum was horrified when I first told her,*' recalls Nicki. '*She said, "I'll have to tell people you had a holiday romance, I can't tell anyone at church." My aunt – who's 17 years younger than her – told her not to be like that, that you can't have secrets around a child. So she did tell her friends, and they were lovely, very supportive.*'

Today, Nicki and her partner, Rosie, have two teenage children, each conceived with sperm from a different donor. Nicki's mum now celebrates Christmas with her extended, unconventional family: Nicki and Rosie, one donor-dad and his wife, the other donor-dad and his companion, and of course the two grandchildren of whom she has become so proud. The relationship between Nicki and her mum has grown stronger as a result. '*Having children has been something that's brought us together,*' reflects Nicki. '*It was something she could relate to.*'

You may get pregnant in a way that your parents don't understand or approve of, like Chantelle. You may find, like Nicki, that your parents don't want to tell people about your family, because they worry what their friends will think. But even if your parents are initially unsure, parenting can become an area of common ground. Your parents may stop talking about their daughter and her 'friend', or about their 'bachelor' son and when he might settle down. Instead they can flash around pictures of the grandchildren to rival anyone else's. They can instruct you how to soothe a teething baby, insist that solid food at four months never did you any harm and give out chocolate before bedtime – in other words, they can say and do to you all the things that their friends say and do to their children.

Coping with conflict

Not every story has a happy ending. Some families might grudgingly accept a relative as LGBT but refuse to accept that they would make a suitable parent. Family ties may not be enough to prevent relationships breaking down. This can be devastating. But, despite the pain, the people we spoke to chose not to focus on broken relationships. Instead, they acknowledged the sadness and hurt, and paid tribute to other relatives and friends who stepped forward with unconditional love.

'*My wife's parents are Turkish, and you might assume would be less accepting, because they live in a country with no LGBT rights and had never heard of two women getting married and making a baby*,' says Hannah, who celebrated the birth of their first child earlier this year. '*On the contrary they couldn't have been more supportive. In fact, members of my own family, who are British, have since disowned me.*

'*It broke my heart to think that our daughter would miss out on one set of grandparents and two uncles. But the biggest loss is to them, for not knowing our amazing little girl. When we take her to Turkey, the love that she receives more than makes up for it, and in the UK we're trying to socialise with other LGBT families so that she will be surrounded by positive and accepting people. It's difficult with our only supportive relations being thousands of miles away, but my wife and I make a strong team and overcome any obstacles together.*'

For some families, relationships can become strained if you come out later in life, after you've had children. Your parents can feel that they are losing the son or daughter they thought they knew. It's especially hard when coming out is linked to the breakdown of a straight relationship and the loss of a partner whom your family liked. Miriam's mother struggled when her daughter first came out as a lesbian. Miriam had been married to her university boyfriend for 11 years and they had a five-year-old daughter. For Miriam, the process of discovering her new lesbian identity, getting a divorce, helping her daughter cope with the changes and negotiating co-parenting with her ex have all gone as smoothly as she could have hoped. But the relationship with her mother is still strained.

'*My mum was in tears when I told her*,' says Miriam remembering the difficult months after she first came out. '*She adored my husband, she still does. It was a complete surprise to her, she couldn't get her head round it. For over a year we hardly* spoke. We just saw each other once a week when I collected my daughter from her after school. We kept it as brief as we could and didn't talk about anything real, just little things about my daughter's day. It was an estrangement of sorts.' But, despite stretching to breaking point, they have come through. They are now able to maintain a functional, if not close, relationship.

Your parents may reject you totally, or they may stay in contact, only to criticise the choices you've made. If this is the case, should you try to preserve the relationship at all costs, or decide to step away for a time? Miriam decided to maintain a relationship with her mother, despite the difficulties, but Rajo, another lesbian mother, made the opposite decision. She's decided that it's best to keep her distance from her mother, for her own well-being and that of her children. She explains: 'My mum doesn't approve of my family. She is vocal about it and very stuck in her ways. She'd like to see the children more often, but I don't think she should, because she has extreme views which are not good for them. She's known for a long time about my sexuality, so have my brothers and sisters. In a way it's a blessing that none of them want to see us, as they would say things which are unhelpful. Life's complicated enough.'

Rajo and her partner, Varinder, each gave birth to one of their children, and Rajo has taken practical steps to ensure that her birth family can't undermine the family that she's created. She and Varinder share legal responsibility for both children, and Rajo's sister-in-law would become the children's guardian in the event of their deaths. 'I wanted to get it done legally because I thought, knowing my luck, my biological family will come along and say they've got rights, because they didn't agree with the family we were bringing the children up in,' she says.

Dealing with questions

You may be the first LGBT parent that your relatives have ever encountered. From your hard-of-hearing great-granny to your curious little nephew, they are bound to have questions. If you treat questions as an opportunity, rather than a source of embarrassment, then your extended family will see same-sex relationships as normal instead of something to be hidden away, and see LGBT parenting as just another way to start a family – and all thanks to you.

Yet it might not be you who faces questions directly. However open you are with your family, some members might feel it's rude to ask you – even if they are desperate to know – so they'll ask another relative instead. To help your family members who find themselves in this situation (and to prevent the gossip), you can prepare them to answer questions correctly and thoughtfully, or to refuse to answer if that's appropriate.

Sally is comfortable talking about her family; she even blogs about her experiences as a non-biological lesbian mum. But there are some questions which family members have never asked her directly, choosing to ask her parents instead. *'No one has ever asked me what our sperm donor looks like, but I know that my aunt, once I had shared our good news, immediately called my parents and asked them',* says Sally. *'She wanted to know his colouring, his build and, no doubt, his intelligence. My parents replied that they didn't know and that it wasn't relevant to them. Full marks!'*

In Dónal's family, the arrival of his two adoptive children sparked conversations within the family: *'The smaller children have asked their parents how two daddies can make a baby, and this was used as an opportunity to explain adoption and homosexuality.'* Dónal never doubted that his large and loving family would welcome his sons as their own. Like many LGBT parents, he is keen to point out that his parents love all their grandchildren equally, regardless of their origins. *'In both our families, the boys are loved and treated exactly the same as biologically born cousins',* he says. *'I had an adopted aunt and my sister is also an adoptive mother. There was never any anti-gay parenting feeling from anyone. Until our boys came home, my mother had only one grandson and was thrilled to have two more.'*

When Bronwen adopted her daughter, she similarly knew her extended family would have questions, especially the younger members. Her daughter was already nine years old when the adoption took place and Bronwen recognised that everyone would need time to get used to this new relationship. So she did her preparation, suggesting ways that family members could explain to their children about her new daughter and how she came to join their family. It paid off. *'My family, both close and wider, has been brilliantly accepting. My daughter arrived as the oldest child in the family and was accepted by all the children, no questions asked! Well, certainly not to her or to myself.'* The proof that she was now truly part of the family? *'We went to a family event and saw her picture on my cousin's toilet wall – in her spot on the family tree.'*

Involving your extended family

It's a cliché, but a true one, that it takes a village to raise a child. Grandparents, or great-grandparents, can dote on and spoil your children. Cousins can become their playmates and peers, and your sisters and brothers, their aunts and uncles, can each have a special role.

Susie found her brother was a great support during the process of transitioning. Not just for her, but for her children too. While she's repeatedly reassured her children that she'll always love them and always be their dad, her ten-year-old son has sometimes found it hard to adjust. *'He was concerned about losing a male role model,'* says Susie. *'My ex-wife tells him that he's the man of the family now. He's come to me, crying, saying that we won't do "dad stuff" – that I won't teach him how to ride a bike or go fishing. I say, "You know how to ride a bike, and we can still go fishing if you want to." It helps that he's able to turn to his uncle, my brother, too. My son can talk to him and ask him questions that he couldn't ask me. My brother has been ace. He doesn't get into the details, he just says he's got a sister now.'*

Susie has a good relationship with her grandparents and knows that age is no barrier to dealing with change. She says, *'My 87-year-old grandma now calls me Susie, she's found my separation with my wife harder to deal with than my transitioning.'* Sometimes older relatives can be *more* open and understanding than younger ones. They've lived through change themselves and can take the long view.

Lesbian mum Jackie has always been close to her aunt Leila, now in her 90s, and appreciates her aunt's down-to-earth attitude to life. '*When I realised Jackie was gay, I didn't have any concerns, but I didn't think she'd have kids,*' says Leila. '*I thought it was a shame that my sister wouldn't have any grandchildren, so I was delighted when Jackie was pregnant. My generation grew up with the idea that being gay is unnatural, it's not something to be talked about. It's so different now, people are so much more open-minded. I'm 95, I've seen changes in everything. It's much better today. To me, it makes no odds what someone's sexuality is.*'

For Jackie, and other single parents, support from extended family members can be particularly important. It can bring the opportunity to forge new and stronger bonds, as well as tensions of its own. '*My immediate family were not that supportive initially,*' admits single parent Bronwen. '*My wanting to adopt came at a time when my parents were both unwell. They were concerned that they wouldn't be there to help me due to the distance between us, and the fact their parents were ageing and needed increasing support. However, when it came to it, they have been very supportive and positive.*'

Lea has been a solo parent from day one, and says, '*I wouldn't know how to cope in a two-parent family. It's normal having to split myself into a million pieces and to do everything myself.*' Yet she also recognises that support from her parents, however much they don't see eye-to-eye on many things, is incredibly important to her. '*My mum comes round most lunchtimes,*' she says, '*and she drives me potty. But when she's away on holiday, I realise I do need her.*'

It's not only single parents that benefit from the support of their parents or extended family. We all come under pressure at times, and that's when being able to call on family members for support is most crucial. But when Rajo and her partner first started trying to get pregnant at a clinic, she had not thought family connections would be necessary. '*I thought our friends would be our family,*' she explains. '*I had no contact with my family because of my sexuality, although my partner is very close to her family.*'

Despite this closeness, Rajo wasn't sure about meeting her partner, Varinder's, family and they decided not to tell them about their plans to have children. '*Varinder didn't want to tell her family for fear they might say that this was not the way to have a child. But gradually she started thinking it would be good to have the family support, and that we should move down to where they are. I thought, Oh, I'm not sure about all this working out.'*

Months went by, and Rajo failed to get pregnant. Then Varinder tried, still no luck. They remained cautious about sharing their plans with the extended family, until a crisis forced their hand: *'Varinder's brother got ill. We temporarily moved in with her family to be closer to him – and much to my surprise I really liked them! A lot of her family live a few doors apart on the same street: two brothers and a sister on the same block. They are a very close family, which took some getting used to. But I said, "If you want to stay, then we can." So we moved down and have always felt this was the right decision.'*

Despite living down the road from Varinder's family, they were each still travelling to the clinic near where they used to live on alternate months, trying and failing to conceive. Then Varinder's mother came up with a better plan: *'She said, "This is really stressful, you go and then she goes, you should both try at the same time." We thought that would be really chaotic, what if we both got pregnant at once? She said, "If it's meant to be, it's meant to be."'*

And it *was* meant to be. *'We both got pregnant the first time we tried together. We were excited for a few minutes, then thought, Oh my god, was this a good idea? We were overwhelmed at the thought of being parents to two children.'* The situation that many lesbian couples wonder or joke about became a reality for Rajo and her partner.

One child is tough enough when you're not used to caring for someone who is so utterly dependent on you. Overnight, your whole world changes, and it never stops changing. The challenge – both practical and emotional – gets much harder if you have two or more children at the same time, for example, giving birth to twins or adopting a sibling group. At these times, we rely on relatives and friends and, for couples, really value a partner's support. But because Rajo and Varinder's babies were due within days of each other, they were limited in how much they *could* physically support each other. This was when the extended family came into its own. Even those of us who love our in-laws deeply, and have shared many things with them, still might be struck by how much Varinder's family supported Rajo and Varinder and helped them to cope.

'*Those last few weeks when we were both heavily pregnant were difficult,*' remembers Rajo. '*When my partner gave birth it was really hard, I was with her in labour and when she had an emergency C section. The hospital knew we were partners and let me stay as late and come as early as they could – but I was absolutely exhausted. The family were a great support then.*

'*Ten days later, when I gave birth, it was very difficult for Varinder to be there. She was breastfeeding and our daughter was very clingy. Her brother, who lives across the street, took me in to the hospital. Her mum was with me the whole time I was in labour. She'd never witnessed the birth of a baby before, and so she formed a really strong bond with our son.*'

Extended family members can offer practical and emotional support, whatever your family structure is like. But, for LGBT families, it matters even more to know that your family affirms your identity and choices, when society may not always do so. Faye, who had children in an opposite-sex marriage before she came out, is grateful for this kind of support from her family, and the down-to-earth wisdom of her grandmother Barbara: '*A child needs happiness,*' says Barbara. "*If you are living life being true to yourself like my granddaughter Faye, then you can create a happy home for a child to grow up in. A family, regardless of gender or sexuality, is about happiness, love and respect.*'

Top tips

1. **Give them time.** If your family's first response is not what you hoped for, take a deep breath and wait. You've probably been thinking and planning parenthood – or preparing to come out if you are already a parent – for a long time before talking to them. Give them time to adjust.

2. **Give them information.** A copy of this book, for example! Suggest that they meet other LGBT parents and their families, through personal contacts or an organisation like Families and Friends of Lesbians and Gays (FFLAG), to ask

the questions they feel they can't ask you directly. You don't have to tell them the ins and outs of the process, unless you want to, but be ready to correct any misconceptions. Answer questions from children in your family honestly and appropriately. A picture book speaks a thousand words, so why not buy them a copy of Mary Hoffman and Ros Asquith's *The Big Book of Families* or Todd Parr's *The Family Book* – adults love these too! If you come from a particular religious background, seek out supportive resources within that tradition to help reassure your family that they can still be good Jews, Christians, Sikhs, Muslims or whatever faith they follow, while being proud of their LGBT family members.

3. **Ask their advice.** Who better to give you parenting advice than your own parents or your big brother or sister who already has their own kids? You don't have to agree with everything they say, but asking for their advice, about coping with morning sickness or sleepless nights, focuses them on what you have in common, rather than the differences.

4. **Make time to mourn.** If there are family members who can't accept you or your children, you may end up losing contact. If you can, give yourself time and space to mourn the ending or changing of those relationships.

5. **Don't make assumptions.** We might think we know our families inside out and can predict their reactions, and often we can. But sometimes they can surprise us, so be open to getting a positive response that you don't expect. Joyfully celebrate the family relationships you have. Every offer of babysitting, every school nativity play attendance, even every bit of advice, is a gift that shows you and your children how much you are loved.

9

OUT AND ABOUT

LGBT families with young children can face questions from all sides: from health visitors, adoption and fostering agencies, midwives and other parents. This chapter helps you to negotiate these encounters; and shares stories that are funny, frustrating and thought-provoking.

Birth, adoption and the early years are the times when families are most under scrutiny. These are also the times when you are at your most clueless as a parent, especially with your first child. Everything is new, the systems in place can be baffling and you may be anxious about what questions people will ask.

You may also experience what lesbian mum Shirley describes as '*the impossible pressure to be seen as perfect*'. She continues, '*I think the main difference between us and a straight family is the dearth of role models. We have been on a long and painful journey to have our beautiful sons. We have to grapple with parental roles and how the outside world views us. We are always wondering what the next stranger will come out with when they see us out and about.*'

The pressure hasn't gone away but, for Shirley and Ailsa, it has got easier. As their sons have got older, they have become more confident and comfortable with their roles as parents and their visibility as an LGBT family: '*We are still learning, but we are definitely becoming more comfortable with the challenge,*' says Shirley. '*We have gone against the grain in so many ways: being a LGBT family, being older parents, having a known dad. It is often hard to find the time to reflect on the miracle that has occurred – day-to-day life can be challenging and tiring. I feel thankful for our wonderful boys and so proud of the family we have created. We remind ourselves that we are trailblazers for the future. That matters.*'

It's wise to be prepared. The birth or adoption placement itself will be the moment when you realise this crazy plan of having children is no longer just a nice idea, but a noisy, messy and sleepless reality. But you start being publicly visible as an LGBT family before you even have a child: at antenatal classes, midwife appointments or throughout the pre-adoption process.

Antenatal classes

As soon as you waddle through the door as a birth mother, and struggle panting into a chair, it's pretty clear what you're doing here. For the non-bio mum, clutching the leaflet entitled 'Dads: What you need to know', it's less so. And it's slightly disconcerting being the only woman in the room without a bump or the need to rush to the loo every ten minutes.

How antenatal classes go depends on many things. Some are to do with the course itself: who's running it and how clued up they are about LGBT families, what material they use and what the other participants are like. Some are to do with you: how anxious you feel about being there, how at ease you feel talking about your family set-up and whether your goal is to make friends for life, or simply to get through the evening.

Despite her initial fears, Clare's experience at antenatal classes was positive. Having just moved from the city to a small town, she was worried about sticking out in the sticks. *'The first health professionals I met assumed not only that I was straight but also married,'* she explains. *'I became worried I was in the wrong place to be a gay parent. What a relief that at our local NCT class of six couples, we not only met another lesbian couple but also an accepting group of people who have become valued friends. This gave us confidence that we are in the right place to bring up our children and that we would be accepted for who, and not what, we are.'*

However, this experience is not shared by everyone. Few people experience hostility at antenatal classes, but same-sex couples have found it hard to fit into such a heterosexual system. It's especially unsettling for non-biological mums trying to work out their roles. Jenny was unsure whether or not to accept the invite to the NCT 'dads' curry night (she didn't). Beth found that, on the hospital tour, the midwife kept referring to what 'Dad' was going to be doing. When she questioned this, the midwife carried on as before, but looked at Beth every time she referred to 'Dad' again. And Ailsa couldn't work out whether to join the mums or dads group in her antenatal classes: she was going to be a mum, yet was also like the dads, there to give her partner the support she needed to give birth.

However much confusion you think you'll encounter attending antenatal classes as a lesbian couple, surely the potential for misunderstanding is far greater for a gay male couple preparing for their surrogate to give birth. And yet Felix and Evan handled it with aplomb. '*We got on with everyone in our NCT group, we still see them all the time*,' says Felix, now father of a three-year-old. '*The facilitator was caught between saying "breast is best", but then, because she wanted to be nice to the gay couple, saying, "Not for you of course, bottle-feeding's fine." Others in the group came to me for bottle-feeding advice because, believe it or not, we didn't breastfeed. The only issue was that we couldn't both be on the mailing list for the dads, the form didn't allow it, so one of us had to be the designated woman.*'

The fostering and adoption process

The process to become an adoptive or foster parent can dominate your life for months, with no guarantee of success. Social workers interview you at home, ask your friends and family for references, and introduce you to other potential adopters or foster carers for training and information sessions.

A year after the law changed to allow same-sex couples to adopt, and over ten years since they had first started planning to have children, Dónal and his partner joined the LGBT fostering and adoption group New Family Social and started trying to find an adoption agency: '*We contacted so many local authorities. It was heartbreaking, as one after the other said that we were the wrong race, too old, or that children needed mothers. One local authority agreed to meet us, but the interview was dreadful. A gay couple we had met through New Family Social suggested a voluntary organisation, because they had had a good experience with them. And they were right, from the get-go this organisation was amazing.'*

But in order to make it through the process, and prove that they would be good parents, they felt that they had to compromise their LGBT identity and their queer activism in subtle, unspoken ways: *'We never discussed it, but in truth, we presented ourselves as mirror images of a heterosexual couple,'* says Dónal, looking back. *'Heteronormative assumptions were made about us and we never corrected them. The assessment process is so intrusive already and, while taking part, all the power lies with the agency, so we felt that during the assessment was not the time to be activists.'*

'*The whole process was beyond anything we could have expected or prepared for,'* agrees Alison, a more recent adopter than Dónal, who has just emerged from the process. *'Over the visits and preparation, we were broken down to the core. We vowed to be the best parents ever at the end of all this,'* she admits. Now, in between changing nappies and dealing with tantrums, she can stop and reflect on her experience. *'All the training was geared towards heterosexual couples,'* she recalls. *'I can understand why, it's only recently that they've "let" us gay people adopt. We were the only same-sex couple in our group. We got the impression we were the only same-sex couple many of the social workers had worked with. We were quite a novelty for them, but we didn't mind.'*

Alison had expected that the training would be designed and delivered with straight couples in mind. What she hadn't expected was how much would be focused on coming to terms with loss. *'For most of the heterosexual couples on the course, exploring loss meant coming to terms with miscarriage, failed IVF or infertility after chemotherapy, meaning they weren't able to have biological children,'* continues Alison. *'We didn't go through that. We didn't feel loss when we prepared to be adoptive parents, we were really excited!'*

As Alison found to her surprise, exploring issues of loss and infertility are part of the adoption assessment process for straight and LGBT prospective parents alike, even those for whom adoption is their first choice. Since gay men and lesbians can have biological children, you may be asked to reflect on why you are pursing adoption, rather than other options.

Andrew and his partner, William, also didn't know what to expect when they went to their first adoption evening. Months of meetings, assessments and ups and downs followed before they adopted their son, but that first evening made a huge impression on them, in particular because the experience of gay male adopters like themselves was explicitly included: '*I vividly remember listening to social workers telling a diverse group of 60+ people what the timelines were and what to expect going through the process,*' says Andrew. '*We saw a video which had two gay dads talking about their experience. This gave us both more positive thoughts that we were doing the right thing.*'

By contrast, Carla is a social worker in a fostering and adoption team herself, which meant she had the advantage of knowing the system inside out before she started her own family through adoption. '*We didn't encounter any issues with being a same-sex couple in the adoption process,*' she says categorically. '*I don't think the fact that we were a same-sex couple was even mentioned when we went to the approval panel. It was more difficult because I was a social worker and because I had been adopted myself.*'

Foster carers Jay and Dee have had a more mixed experience with social workers, but aren't afraid to challenge inappropriate behaviour when it occurs: '*Our original social worker asked too many questions about us as a same-sex couple. Short of asking what we did in the bedroom, he asked pretty much everything else,*' says Jay. '*In the feedback, I said we'd found this inappropriate. He was very honest, he said we were the first same-sex couple he'd assessed and he wanted to cover everything. We told him, it shouldn't be any different from assessing a man and a woman. He apologised, but we came across this kind of thing a few times from social workers.*'

During the birth

As with antenatal classes, perinatal services are not always set up to deal with same-sex couples. Even the smoothest birth will be one of life's most emotionally and physically intense experiences. In all the joy and anxiety of the birth and first few days, you might not have much time or energy to reflect on what happened until much later.

While the vast majority of births in the UK and Ireland take place in hospitals or birthing centres, a growing number of women opt to give birth at home. For LGBT families this means being confident to welcome professionals into your home, but also means that you are not in a strange environment and have more say over what happens during the birth and the aftermath, including who can be there, than you would in a hospital. For mum of two Jessica, this was a very positive experience. She explains, *'We have had overwhelmingly good relationships with the professionals who have come into our lives since having our kids – with one or two glaring exceptions. Doctors, midwives, NCT practitioners... all lovely. We had two home births and both times had amazing support. Our midwives were phenomenal and I loved having a choccy biscuit and cup of tea with them to celebrate each of our safe arrivals.'*

Marie and Beth, Nicki and Rosie, and Felix and Evan are all same-sex couples who had negative or mixed experiences giving birth in hospitals. But each of these experiences, which they share below, made them more determined to assert their roles and to seek out mutual support from other LGBT parents.

Beth had already felt sidelined as a non-biological mum during antenatal classes, so she and her partner, Marie, took a special effort to be well-prepared for the birth: *'We'd written a birth plan, and carefully included about our relationship, even who was going to be "mummy" and who was "mama",* says Beth. *'They didn't read it. The birth was long and difficult. Several staff members that came in asked me, "Who are you? Where's her husband?" They didn't even phone me when Marie went into the birthing suite from the prenatal ward. They were under-resourced and that was one of the impacts. At the time we kept saying, "It's fine, it's fine" – but looking back, we can say it was rubbish.'*

They've now had time to reflect on and come to terms with that experience, and advise other couples to be prepared. *'As a non-birth mum, you need to be resilient. You need to actively claim your role and prepare for it to be undermined,'* advises Marie. *'In the middle of giving birth is not a great time to be able to defend your partner's rights, so work out as a couple in advance how you're going to deal with this.'*

Rosie and Nicki have two children, now secondary school age. How Rosie has been treated as a non-biological mum has shaped her determination to claim her role. *'For me, it's been about feeling equal, claiming my part,'* she says. *'We've all got our internalised homophobia which can make it hard to do. When Nicki was in hospital after giving birth, they wouldn't let me in the ward, they wouldn't believe I was her partner. You have to be pretty strong, surrounded by all these husbands, to say, "I am her partner."'*

It's not just lesbian parents who have to negotiate the hospital system. As Felix and Evan found out, *'being a gay male couple dealing with the NHS in a bit of Britain where they've never heard of surrogacy is a challenge'.* Despite speaking to the hospital many times in advance, Felix and Evan found the practical boundaries were hard to get around. Evan explains, *'It wasn't so much because we were a gay couple, but because we were men. There was no place they could guarantee we'd be able to stay for the night. They couldn't have men on the ward, and if it was a busy night they couldn't guarantee there'd be a private room available. We said we had to be there to care for our baby straight after he was born.'*

'I think they were terrified,' chips in Felix. *'It had never happened for men to be in charge of babies in that unit before. It felt like they were more concerned about not fucking up than about doing the right thing by us. Next time, it will be totally different. I'll be less in awe. We'll work it through earlier with the hospital and get references from other hospitals.'*

But in the end, their worries about not being able to care for their son immediately after birth were replaced by different worries. *'He was born so early that we only got to hold him briefly before he was taken to the intensive care unit,'* says Felix. *'We had heard terrible stories about when babies go into the ICU, one hospital that insisted only the surrogate could take the baby out of the incubator and then give the baby to the dads. We never encountered anything like that. To be honest, from the moment they realised we were the dads – all the rules went out of the window. We had the most amazing care.'*

Coming out, day in, day out

LGBT parents are everywhere. But many people have still never encountered a real-life LGBT family. When they do, they can be surprised, intrigued or full of questions. '*When you've been out for a while you get used to not having to come out,*' explains lesbian mum Victoria. '*But now that I'm a parent, not a day goes by without having to come out to someone. Mostly it's fine, but I do find it tiring. It even happened when we moved house. Our new neighbour knocked on our door to say hi, but, when she realised we were two women with a child, she was so surprised that she had to go back home and compose herself. She came back five minutes later to apologise. We're on good terms now. Most people soon realise you are just as dull as they are.*'

Once you have a baby, people you don't know stop and talk to you all the time, in shops, streets or public transport. They comment on the baby's gender or admire its outfit, ask if it looks more like you or like your husband/wife, or simply take the opportunity to pass on unasked-for parenting advice. Pushing a pram around a park can have the same effect as wearing a sign saying, 'Talk to me (oh, and by the way don't hold back on any personal questions)'. It's as sociable as having a dog.

Jenny and her female partner have two young children and they'll often take it in turns to go out and about with the kids. Jenny's happy to chat to anyone she meets in the park or the playground, but sometimes it can get awkward. '*There's a woman I see in the park with a little girl. The last time I saw her was months ago when she was heavily pregnant,*' says Jenny. '*I recently saw her again, so I went over to see the baby and say "hello". We hadn't really spoken before. She replied that she'd seen my children at the playground recently with their mother.*'

Those of us who are lesbian or gay parents will recognise this kind of situation. Where you are assumed to be a childminder or an aunt instead of a mother. Or where you are commended for looking after the kids while your wife has a break, when your husband's standing right next to you. Is it always worth the bother – and potential awkwardness – of coming out?

Jenny continues, '*I thought, One, who do you think I am then? and two, should I go into it? And then I thought, Oh, I can't be bothered. I meet people in the park all the time, and they just assume I'm heterosexual. Most of the time I have to clarify who I am at some point in the conversation. So I'll drop into the conversation "my partner, Lucy", or "they have two mums", or something like that. I don't know why I do that – maybe to gauge their reaction or, if they've got a problem with it, I'll know not to speak to them again!'*

Once your children get older however, it's no longer a question of how prepared you are to come out, but how quickly they'll out you anyway. Father of two Dónal is getting used to this experience: *'As an adoptive queer father, I am often amazed that people feel entitled to interrogate me about our boys' past: "Why were they in care? What happened to them at home? Who are their parents? Are they related? When do you have to return them?" Often people make comments to the children about their mother, assuming that she's waiting at home. Once, when I was particularly stressed because of the boys' challenging behaviour in a shopping centre, a helpful woman assured me that I now knew what my wife had to deal with on a daily basis. The boys thought this was hilarious and told the woman that I didn't have a wife, I didn't even have a husband, as I wasn't married to Papa. The look on her face was priceless.'*

Sometimes when you come out about being an LGBT parent, you don't know whether you are going to be judged, interrogated or congratulated. Thankfully, with recent social and legal changes in the UK and Ireland, negative reactions are becoming rarer. But, as lesbian mum Kim found, when they come, it's all the more shocking and upsetting for being unexpected. *'We saw a locum GP for a routine health check a week after our son was born,'* explains Kim. *'The GP asked us a lot of questions about how our son was conceived, which led on to a lecture about how confused he will be later in life and how having a lot of half-siblings due to donor conception will cause issues for him. This was the first time I had left the house with my new baby and I came out of the appointment in tears. We made a formal complaint to the GP surgery who handled it very well.'*

At the other extreme, some people are delighted to meet LGBT families, giving us kudos and congratulations just for existing. '*We have only encountered positive reactions,*' says Sophie. '*People seem ready for change and keen to embrace a more open-minded and tolerant society. We have, oddly, on more than one occasion, even been congratulated for being in a civil partnership and having a child together!*'

To prove that our families are just as valid as anyone else's, we risk piling pressure on ourselves to get it right all the time. There's a voice, however faint, in the back of our minds, whispering that everyone's waiting for us to fail. While this is not just paranoia – the Irish marriage referendum's 'No' campaign, anti-gay religious groups and the tabloid media have all made use of scare stories about the damaging impact of LGBT parenting – it's not the whole truth either. However tough things are, there will be someone on your side – your mum, your brother, your LGBT friends, your children's teacher or your kids themselves – to whom you have nothing to prove. They know what a great job you're doing and, if you're very lucky, will even tell you so too.

Adoptive mum Carla sums it all up with a down-to-earth reminder: '*Without sounding too twee, I've not had negative experiences of parenting or of people's attitudes. Sometimes we get hung up on stuff that isn't there. People are just people. Just get on and be a family.*'

Top tips

1. **Find out and feedback.** If you're worried before an appointment or a class, you can phone the organisers in advance to find out what experience they have of LGBT parents or to explain about your family set-up. Afterwards, if you think they could have better catered for the needs of LGBT parents, then let them know. It may not affect you after the fact, but constructive feedback can change how classes are run or how staff behave in the future, so others can benefit from your experience.

2. **Educate.** You may be the first LGBT family that other parents-to-be, your midwife or social worker have met. People aren't usually hostile to LGBT families, they just don't know any. Take the opportunity to educate. Not necessarily by drawing a diagram of your family tree or

giving a step-by-step guide to home insemination, but by being friendly and approachable.

3. **Keep it in proportion.** You hear of parents who meet at antenatal classes and still meet up for weekly coffees (or gins) when their children are grown up. These relationships can be an enormous support and source of friendship. Or not. You don't have to sign up for life. You don't have to ever see these people again, and that's okay too. The same is true for any baby group, class or social activity, difficult social worker or insensitive midwife.

4. **Talk to other LGBT prospective parents.** Groups like New Family Social are invaluable for those considering adoption or going through the process, as well as for those who have emerged out the other side. Some adoption agencies even pay for your membership as part of the adoption support package. In chapter 15 'Staying gay', you can find more about the support available for all kinds of LGBT families.

10

SCHOOL'S OUT

From the ages of 4 to 18, most children spend thousands of hours of their lives at school. So do parents – with parents' evenings, Christmas fairs and the daily school run. This chapter explores what it's like being an LGBT family in the school system, including how to choose a school and assess if it is LGBT-friendly; and advises on how to build a good relationship with the school.

Many of us haven't been back to school since we picked up our exam results years ago. The noise, the smell, the feel of the place, once so familiar, is now a vague memory. It's even longer since we first started school, yet now we're back at the beginning. This time we don't even get to do any finger-painting or make castles out of papier mâché. We have become the anxious parents, catapulting our children into this mysterious world beyond our view, where they will spend most of their waking hours until they are almost adults themselves.

Unless you are a teacher or work closely with schools, you may not realise what has changed in recent years concerning how different families, and LGBT issues in general, are discussed and valued in schools. The casual use of homophobic language is still startlingly common. Some children are still bullied because of their gender non-conformity, perceived sexual orientation or family structure. Not all schools are confident in dealing with such bullying when it occurs, and even fewer go out of their way to stop it occurring, despite the legal requirement to do so. There is still a long way to go. But the legacy of Section 28, which prohibited schools from 'promoting the teaching of the acceptability of homosexuality as a pretended family relationship', seems to be finally fading.

Many LGBT parents are pleasantly surprised about how well their family has been accepted by teachers, parents and pupils at school. They have not just been silently tolerated, but positively affirmed. Gay dad Scott sums up his experience, *'When our children first started at the school, there was a little suspicion. When we proved over time that we would fight for what we believed in, we gained respect from the head teacher. Fast forward eight years and we are still the only male same-sex couple to have children in the school, but we are respected and our advice is even sought on issues to do with vulnerable children. LGBT families have been visible for such a short time. So while there may not yet be 100 per cent acceptance in all schools, we are getting there.'*

Choosing a school

All families have many different reasons for choosing a school: personal connections, academic, musical or sporting reputation, a faith basis – or whether it's near enough that you can oversleep, leave late, forget your lunchbox, run back to get it and still get to school (just about) on time. For LGBT families in particular, how the school handles diversity and deals with homophobic bullying are also likely to be crucial factors.

Many LGBT parents decide to talk with teachers at potential schools about their family structure before deciding whether to apply to that school, or arrange to meet their child's teacher before term starts. This gives you the opportunity to ask or answer any questions, explain how you want to be referred to and ensure that any homophobic bullying or name-calling will be dealt with.

'School was a worry for us before our daughter started,' admits lesbian mum Mich. When their daughter was born, Mich and her partner lived in a gay-friendly area of a large city. Lots of their friends were same-sex couples with children and their daughter grew up knowing plenty of families like hers. Then, before starting primary school, they moved out of town. They didn't expect the village school to have encountered LGBT families before, and were anxious about the response they would get. *'We didn't know when we applied, but we soon found out that there were other lesbian mums there,'* recalls Mich. *'We explained to the Reception teacher about our daughter having two mummies, and she said: "Oh yeah, we've had that before."*

So far, among the same-sex parents we know, there have not been any negative experiences of school or nursery, and that has lessened our worries.'

Jenny and Lucy didn't choose their children's school on the basis of there being other lesbian parents there. They live in an area where there are plenty of LGBT families, so it wouldn't be unreasonable to expect to bump into one or two in the school playground. Even so, when it did happen, it still took them by surprise. *'During our son's first term at school, I suddenly clocked that one of his friends also had two mums,'* Jenny says. *'We said to him, "Does anyone else in your class have two mums?" He didn't know. One of the other mums asked her little girl the same question. She hadn't noticed either. Neither of them knew about each other and when they did they weren't bothered. They had no idea how exciting this was for us.'*

Being part of a minority, even a very small one, is better than being the only one. Even if you only exchange an occasional smile with another LGBT parent when you pass in the playground, it can provide support and solidarity. It also takes the pressure off. It's reassuring to know that the school has had to think about these issues before – it's not up to you alone to fly the flag for LGBT families.

By contrast, the school Victoria and her partner have chosen for their son has no experience of LGBT parents at all. Are they daunted? Not at all. *'It is a very sweet school, but quite conservative,'* explains Victoria. *'We've been in a few times already, including for a tour with the head master. We stuck out like a sore thumb as the only same-sex couple there. Our son is starting soon and the school has begun to ask us lots of things, like "what shall we call you?" I think we'll write the story down for them, so they know what our son knows. We'll talk it through as well, but if we write it down then it's there for all the staff to see.'*

A supportive head teacher is very important, but it's not always enough, as Nicki and Rosie found out in their chosen school. *'When we spoke to the head she was very positive,'* remembers Nicki. *'She told us that she had a gay brother, but that she didn't know of any other gay families in the school. She did order Stonewall posters, but the teachers wouldn't put them up.'* Their experience with individual teachers at the school was mixed.

Nicki and Rosie never kept their family structure a secret at their children's primary school. It wouldn't have worked anyway. *'In year four, our daughter explained to her whole class how she was made,'* remembers Rosie. *'She told them about her donor-dad shaking his willy to get the semen, and then bringing it in a syringe on a motorbike, so that I could put it into Nicki. We heard about it all from another parent, who thought it was really funny.'* Even before the class found out about the ins and outs of home insemination, the teacher had been good at integrating mentions of same-sex families into lessons. But other teachers were determined to avoid the issue entirely, however relevant it might be: *'There was one who taught the class about the Holocaust. I asked her whether she'd talked about how gay people had been killed in the Holocaust. "No," she said, "we don't talk about homosexuals. If a word has 'sex' in it, the children will only giggle."'*

Keeping the faith

Lesbian mum Carla was brought up as a Christian, although now describes her faith as *'dented by my experience of homophobia in different churches'*. And yet she chose to send her children to a faith school. Why? *'We chose it because it was the best in the area to meet their needs. They are adopted, so we could choose any school in the country if we wanted! When we phoned our school to ask to look round, we said: "We are a same-sex couple – is this going to be an issue?" The head teacher called us back, horrified that we had to ask. She seemed gobsmacked that we would think this could be a problem. We don't feel we've been treated differently from any of our children's friends' parents. We've not had any bad experiences.'*

Organised religion doesn't have a good reputation for affirming or celebrating LGBT people and their families. Which is why even LGBT parents who are religious themselves might have concerns about sending their children to a faith school. Bronwen's Christian faith is important to her. When her daughter changed schools shortly after being adopted, Bronwen deliberately chose a church school, but remained concerned about how they were going to teach sex education. *'I went to the parents' meeting and specifically asked how they were teaching LGBT family values,'* she says. *'My question was answered in a very positive light of acceptance.'*

Bronwen followed up her public question with a private conversation with her daughter's class teacher. *'I let her know that I was a lesbian and told her that my daughter knew,'* says Bronwen, also explaining to the teacher that she had advised her daughter not to discuss this with her friends. *'She has more than enough to be dealing with – and for other kids to have a go at her about – without adding her new mum's sexuality to the mix.'* The class teacher supported her decision and Bronwen left the meeting satisfied.

Some parents believe that faith schools can be better places for children in LGBT families than secular alternatives. *'Our older son attends a Church of England primary school,'* says Heather. *'Before he started, we went to see two schools. When we told one of the head teachers about our situation, she said, "Well, we have families of all types here. There are lots of families where there is no dad." I felt she had missed the point – that homophobic bullying is a real possibility for our children and we wanted the school to look out for that. The head teacher of the Church of England school, on the other hand, seemed to get it. She assured us that they would be mindful of his family relationships. They have been true to their word. I was worried about him going to a faith school, but actually the value base they promote means the environment feels safer.'*

Jackie worked in a Jewish school while she was bringing up her son and her partner's son. At first, she was reluctant to come out at school because she feared that, if the news spread in their small community, the children would face prejudice. Yet as more lesbian and gay families started bringing their children to the school and she took on the role of delivering training on homophobic bullying, she didn't want to stay in the closet any longer. *'I spoke to some gay dads before they brought their kids into the school,'* Jackie remembers. *'Unbeknown to me, they deemed us the school of choice for lesbian and gay parents. These men – wow – they were so honest, so visible. Soon after that that I came out to my head teacher.'* Jackie remains proud of what she, the parents and the school achieved together. *'We were the first Jewish primary school to become a Stonewall School Champion,'* she says. *'I was so happy to be making a real difference.'*

While some parents opt for faith schooling, others, like Dónal, don't have much choice. *'Most schools in Ireland are faith-based. In our small town, all the schools are Roman Catholic,'* he says. *'We had no problem getting the boys enrolled and the school has been fairly welcoming. Being atheists has been a bigger issue than us being gay fathers. We struggle with the level of exposure the boys have to the dogma of an organisation that regards us as intrinsically disordered. As far as the school is aware, we are the only LGBT parents (hard to believe in a school of almost 400 kids). That hasn't been an issue, but equally they have been reluctant to do much work on family diversity.'*

Every school, faith-based or secular, has its own value base or philosophy that influences the children they educate. Some are more explicit about this than others. Chantelle has chosen to send her daughter to a Steiner school, which has an alternative approach to education, despite the fact no one else from their local area goes to the school. *'All the kids she plays with at home go to the same, local school,'* says Chantelle. *'She gets on great with them, but also has a completely different group of friends at the Steiner school and experiences a more open-minded environment. There are numerous gay families at the school. It's not an issue, and that's important to me.'*

Some people are gay, get over it:
LGBT families and secondary school

Just when you think you've got it sorted, it's time to start secondary school. It's different this time. Although you are still involved in choosing the school, turning up at parents' evenings and encouraging (or nagging) your children to do their homework, your child has to negotiate their path through secondary school for themselves. By this stage they will also have their own views about how 'out' they want to be about their family at school or among their friends, and their views may differ from yours.

Cathy and her partner, Maz, have brought up their 11-year-old granddaughter since she was little. Now, just about to start secondary school, she remains fiercely proud of her family. *'She's got a rainbow flag up in her window and all sorts,'* says Cathy. *'She's grown up with it, it's all she's ever known, and she's very protective of us.'* Cathy wondered if they'd be able to find a school that would affirm their family, but luck was on their side. *'The day we visited the secondary school was Comic Relief day, so all the kids were in their own clothes,'* she explains. *'I spotted that one of them was wearing a T-shirt saying "Some people are gay, get over it". I asked the head mistress and she told me they have a student-run LGBT group there. She said that they talk about being LGBT and that the school is inclusive. I hadn't come across anything like that in a school round here before, gay people are generally accepted but it's not talked about. I think that this school will be really good for her.'*

There are secondary schools, like the one Cathy visited, which make a real effort to make children with LGBT families feel welcome. Milly, who has two mums, has recently successfully made the transition to secondary school. Her new school shows its commitment to diversity both by tackling bullying and by promoting positive messages. *'When I chose my secondary school, I didn't want to go to a school that had a lot of bullying,'* she says. *'The school I go to has "Some people are gay, get over it" posters up. I knew that before I went there, because my brother's there already. I don't make a big deal of having gay parents, and no one else makes a big deal of it either.'*

Rajo's children are now both 13, forging friendships at secondary school and working out how and when to talk about their family. While giving them all the support she can, Rajo knows that she doesn't have all the answers. She's also having to learn as she goes along.

'Our daughter worries that people might not want to be her friend if they know she has two mums,' says Rajo. *'I try to say that if they don't want to be her friend because of that, then they don't really appreciate her friendship. At the school, they are very good at promoting different families, they have the posters up, they do anti-homophobia campaigns. In Citizenship, they learn about sexism, racism and homophobia, and in the discussions she witnesses some extreme opinions from her peers.*

She watches a lot of documentaries and is acutely aware of prejudice. Our son just gets on with things. His response to any issue is, "Yeah? So? Tough, if they don't like it!"'

While Rajo wants to help her children work out their friendships, and occasionally wants to storm into school and sort it all out herself, she knows that there are lessons they have to learn themselves over time. She tells them, *'If people don't like you, what can you do? It's hard, I know that, but you need to be yourself, sooner rather than later.'*

We're here, we're queer and we're on the PTA

Choosing the right school is important, but it's only the start. Working your way through the school system as an LGBT family can raise questions and challenges at every stage – both for the family and for the school. It can challenge you to think about the kind of education your children are getting and how LGBT-inclusive it really is. It can prompt you to ask questions like: when studying authors, scientists or historical figures who are LGBT, how is this acknowledged and discussed in the classroom? Do textbooks, storybooks or other resources show all kinds of families, so that no one is invisible? Does sex and relationships education adequately and appropriately cover LGBT issues? If a school is open to these questions, or already asking these questions themselves, it's a good sign that this is a place where LGBT families can feel that they truly belong.

However, school is not just about what is taught in the classroom. It's also about the relationships between staff, parents and students. In primary school, the school community includes parents much more than at secondary school, where friendships between pupils and the desire to fit in and be accepted become increasingly significant. Schools – as well as parents and pupils themselves – have to grapple with what this means for children whose families may be seen as unusual or different from the norm.

Schools can vary enormously in their attitudes to LGBT parents, as Katharine found out. From the start, she felt that her son's primary school did not know how to deal with a parent who was trans. However, she only ran into difficulties when his behaviour at school became increasingly challenging. *'I felt they were using me being trans as the hook on which to hang his issues,* she says. *'They weren't exploring other possibilities. It was the only thing which mattered to them. They didn't look into the possibility of Asperger's or learning difficulties or ADHD.'* Katharine fought hard for her son's problems to be assessed. *'Even the professionals involved in the assessment of needs seemed to want to ask extremely personal questions about my situation, or made assumptions that had to be strongly challenged, before they began to see my son in his own light.'*

When Katharine moved her son to a new school, it couldn't have been more different. *'All the staff at the school know I'm trans. It's never been an issue. I have never spoken about it with staff and they have never asked,'* she continues. *'I've just become a parent-governor because the head master strong-armed me into it. I would never have dreamed to put myself forward. It's interesting to see the school from the other side.'*

As parents, our past experiences of school can make it hard to shake off the awkwardness we might feel about being different. It can be a mix between wanting to fit in with other parents in the playground, and a defiant I-don't-care-what-they-think-of-me attitude. *'I've definitely felt isolated in the school playground, I get looks and I know they're talking about me,'* says Mel, who has moved home and school with her daughters more than once since she came out, partly because of the homophobia she's faced. She continues, *'Despite this, there is a group of mums at my younger daughter's school who've been very kind and have included me in evenings out or other meet-ups. I've never experienced that before.'*

One way to enable pupils, parents and staff alike to see LGBT parents as positive role models, and members of the school community just like anyone else, is to get in there. There are lots of ways to get involved. Simply express an interest and you'll be pounced upon. No one's going to care what you do in bed – as long as you offer to help out with the tombola or volunteer to listen to six-year-olds practising their reading.

'Being around at the primary school has been great for visibility of trans people in general,' believes Susie, whose youngest child is just finishing year six. *'The parents are the kind of people who wouldn't want a trans person near their*

children, yet at school I'm seen as just like any other parent. I volunteer for things at school, I even go in and take photos for them. I think once the "think of the children" angle is dealt with, lots of the concern about trans people fades.'

LGBT teachers can also play a positive role in normalising LGBT people and relationships, if they have support from the school. Naomi is pansexual, and both a parent and a teacher. Like Susie, her presence in the classroom provides an opportunity for conversation and gentle challenge, education in its widest sense, to take place. She remembers one instance: *'I was working with a group on the computers at school and we saw a story on a news site about the Equal Marriage Act, along with a picture of two men kissing. There were lots of "eurghs" from the boys who saw the picture, but we talked about it and we got past it. Some just didn't know that two men could get married – and now they do.'*

Mother's Day and Father's Day

If you've got a child in nursery or primary school there's one thing you can be certain of: there are going to be glittery, hand-painted cards. But who will they be addressed to? If there are two dads, should there be just one Father's Day card or two? If there's no dad, who gets the lovingly crafted card? Many families have one parent or have step-parents, so schools should have thought about how to meet the needs of different families. If you think the school won't be sure what to do, you can hope they ask. But the best thing to do is to tell them. It gives you a chance to talk about how your family works, and to avoid any awkwardness or misunderstanding. The main thing is that your child can affirm the people who are important in their life and doesn't feel left out of a class activity.

There are plenty of creative solutions. Carla's children, who have two mums, bring home two Mother's Day cards each from school and nursery. As there's no dad, on Father's Day they give their godfathers a card. Milly, who has two mums, has just moved up to secondary school but, when at primary school, she worked out her own strategy: *'I'd make two cards for Mother's Day, or one card with two names in. For Father's Day I'd make a card but not give it to anyone. I'd tell the teachers*

– sometimes I found it annoying but mostly it was okay.'

Mich was a little surprised when, after dropping her daughter at nursery, one of the staff asked to have a word: *'The staff member looked really anxious, and I wondered what had happened, had my daughter done something wrong? Then she explained that they were doing Father's Day cards. They didn't want her to miss out, but didn't know what she should put on the card. I was really casual about it; I said it's okay to put "Mummy Mich". I could see that she really wanted to get it right and was worried about doing the wrong thing. It was nice that she didn't just assume it would be right to put "father" on the card.'*

It's not just around Mother's Day and Father's Day that such difficulties can occur. Some schools will assume that all families have a mummy and daddy who live together, and it shows in the way in which they communicate with parents. Tony, who came out after his son was born, found that once he and his wife had split up, the school ignored his parental role. *'If your child has both a mother and father the school automatically communicates with the mother,'* he says. *'I was cut out of all dialogue, despite repeatedly asking to be included. It is without doubt one of the most heteronormative institutions I've had to deal with. Thank goodness my ex and I get on, but this is not the case for many.'*

It's not easy to know when to challenge and when to let something lie, especially when you're trying to build a positive relationship with the school. Tony sums up the dilemma: *'If a school doesn't visibly advertise its LGBT policy or support and talks in a heteronormative manner, you either have to challenge or shut up. Neither is conducive to a healthy two-way relationship between the school and the family. My experience has been that the system is not designed for anything other than a standard definition nuclear family.'*

That was Poppy's experience too, when she read through the 'starting school' leaflet that arrived for her son which outlined how 'his mummy and daddy could help him learn at home'. She was concerned, not just because the leaflet disregarded the existence of LGBT families like hers, but it also failed to recognise single-parent households or other kinds of family. She decided to challenge it, and tried to book an appointment with the head teacher. Unfortunately, she was fobbed off. The school told her no one else had complained, and she was just causing trouble. Not a good start to school life.

Managing change

Things change. Some parents split up and some start new relationships. Some come out. Some transition. Families move to new areas and children to new schools. Older adopted or foster children may start new schools when they move in with their new families. There are many reasons why having just one conversation when your child first starts school won't be enough, especially if you think the teachers haven't understood the first time. Any change that may affect our children's ability to learn and thrive, or leave them open to bullying, needs to be addressed in partnership with the school.

It's tough settling into a new school with an older child, when everyone else already knows each other. It's even tougher for a foster child with complex needs. This was a much bigger issue for foster carers Dawn and Paula than being a lesbian couple. *'No one talks to you at the school gates, the other parents don't know what to do with you, you are not part of the community,'* says Dawn. *'You have to be discreet about being foster carers. Our foster son couldn't go round to someone's house for tea, as that would reveal he couldn't be left alone with another child. He couldn't make friends. It's sad really. We were all isolated. Our parents were concerned that, if we had children, they'd be bullied at school for having gay parents. But our little guy was teased for being ginger, not because he had two mums.'*

Justine's family faced a major change when two of her children were still in primary school, as she started to explore transitioning from male to female. Justine and her wife, Julie, decided first to tell their children, and then to tell the school. *'We told the kids before we told anyone else,'* Justine remembers. *'We were honest and explained it to them in plain English. We were clear – it's not a perversion, it's not like what you might have seen on TV. We told them they could come to us if they had any questions, but they were very matter-of-fact about it all.'*

Justine and Julie wanted to tell the school quickly, in case of bullying. The town in northern Scotland where they live is very religious, with traditional gender roles. There's no visible LGBT community. Justine and Julie did not know what the reaction would be, and they expected the worst. Justine continues, *'People can say things in school as a way of hurting someone. Some children would repeat something their parents said, others would use it to hurt our children. It really got to our son. He spoke to his sister about it, although he often wouldn't want to tell us, because he didn't want to upset us. But the school was brilliant. They responded in a good way despite the fact they hadn't come across anyone trans before.'*

Justine's daughter, Samantha, now grown up and a parent herself, agrees. *'The school had no knowledge about trans people, but they bent over backwards to make sure my family and I were protected,'* she says. Life for Samantha as a teenager with a trans parent wasn't easy, but she always knew the school was on her side. *'I was bullied and had to be taxied to and from school to keep me safe,'* she remembers. *'It was horrific. I'd never want to live it again and I'd never wish it on anyone. But any time I needed to speak to someone, I could. I will always be grateful to the school. They made sure I didn't come to any harm. They did the best they could.'*

After divorcing and moving to a new area with her children, Mel's experience of homophobia left her feeling vulnerable and very protective of her children. After she settled both her children in new schools, she had to help them adjust to yet another, happier change, but one which still had its challenges. From being a single parent, Mel now had a female partner. *'I don't think the teacher knows how to handle me, I can sense that awkwardness, she's not sure what to say,'* says Mel. *'So when I told the school I'd got a partner, in case my daughter started mentioning her, I expected the worst. But I was pleasantly surprised that they were fine about it.'*

From inside the classroom

Jess, Bryony and Shoshana come from different backgrounds and their families formed in different ways. But they are all in their twenties now and grew up with lesbian parents at a time when this was less common or socially acceptable than it is today. However, as Shoshana is keen to point out, they are not the only ones. '*There are hundreds of us who have grown up in LGBT+ families and lived to tell the tale,*' she says. '*And we not even close to being in the first generation of children with LGBT+ parents.*'

When they started school, Section 28 was alive and well. By the time they had finished, civil partnerships were legal. Their experiences give an insight into what it's like being at school when you come from an LGBT family, as well as how much has changed in recent years.

'*My parents were worried when I first started school, as they weren't sure that they would be accepted,*' explains Jess. '*LGBT parenting was rarely heard of in the early 90s, and other parents wouldn't understand who the "other woman" was who picked me up from school! At parents' evenings, some teachers wanted to know "who the mother was". It was the first time that I realised my family was different. I don't remember any prejudice at primary school. I don't think that my classmates were old enough to understand what LGBT meant, and we never had any issues from other parents.*'

When Bryony's mum and dad split up, she and her mum moved in with her mum's new female partner, Sue, who became Bryony's other mum. '*I changed primary schools when I was nearly seven years old, at the point when our new family unit was established,*' she recalls. '*I remember my parents deciding against one school because the head teacher got "confused" about our set-up and made some unpleasant comments. I went to a small, multi-cultural, inner-city school. My friends were mostly Asian, some of whom had little or no English, and I was very happy there. Sue still comments that she was more accepted by the Asian mothers at school events than by any of the white parents.*'

However, it wasn't always easy maintaining friendships. Bryony became very aware of people's attitudes, even from an early age, as she explains: '*It was always a delicate balance of ensuring that the friend was fine with it, and then finding out if the parents were. Although they usually were, I had one close friend in primary school who knew, but never told her parents, as they were devoutly religious and very homophobic. As a result, I never did anything with her outside school.*'

Shoshana's parents were always open with her school. *'When I was little, everyone at school knew. My parents would always explain the family set-up to any new school, and my class teachers were fully on board. I guess that when I was five I assumed that there was nothing particularly abnormal about my family,'* she says.

At a time when LGBT families were much less common, the main issue Bryony, Jess and Shoshana faced was the invisibility of families like theirs, and of LGBT people in general, at school. *'There was very little awareness of LGBT issues at all when I was at school,'* says Jess. *'They were not included in sex education classes or mentioned in other lessons. Very little was done to tackle homophobia. A few times, I was bullied and labelled as a "lesbian" because my parents were. I went to see teachers about this, but not much was done. I think awareness of LGBT families has increased massively since I left school. Many of my teachers defined themselves as LGBT, but were not out to the pupils. Sometimes I felt that being LGBT must be embarrassing and that is why they were covering it up.'*

For Bryony, invisibility spilled over into secrecy. She felt pressured not to mention her family at all: *'I was told by teachers in no uncertain terms to not talk about my family, so only my very close friends ever knew. The secrecy felt wrong and was hard to maintain. Neither my primary nor my secondary school did anything at all to tackle homophobia or introduce LGBT role models. I don't think they had to in those days. They certainly did a good job of avoiding it, if they did. I felt fine talking to my close friends about my family, especially once they had been round our house and spent time with us. But if I mentioned it to other children it felt very daring and was often met with fits of giggles or a barrage of abuse.'* But this invisibility and secrecy was not universal: *'I was home-educated for a few years in my teens, and went to a small school for a couple of days a week which was very different. I was in a very small class with two of my close friends, so my family was immediately "outed" and the teachers made sure that this was accepted. My sixth form college had an LGBT society and I joined it.'*

Her advice to children growing up in LGBT families now is simple: *'Now that there is more encouragement for schools to deal with homosexuality positively, I would recommend today's children to be open about their families. They may not be the most popular kids in class as a result, but there will be at least one or two children who are fine with it. They are the people who will make good friends. Who cares about the rest? Have faith that you will meet more open-minded people when you're older.'*

There's a lot to be said for the politicians who repealed Section 28 in the early 2000s and introduced the Equalities Act in 2010; for the activist groups who train and resource schools to help them meet their statutory duties; for the teachers who refuse to endorse a culture of secrecy and shame. But there is another group to thank for improving attitudes to LGBT families in schools. Every child like Shoshana, Jess or Bryony who has been through the school system in previous decades has made it that little bit easier for children of LGBT families today to flourish at school. Their courage has helped LGBT families to become more familiar and so more understood.

As Shoshana puts it, *'I remember being in the playground aged around seven. A lot of kids were curious about the technicalities of lesbians having children. It was a question that could get aggressive. I hadn't quite perfected my scientific answer, but was impressed when Seb, another child of lesbian mothers, explained the turkey baster method in full. That satisfied everyone. The other children were simply curious. Gay parenting wasn't something they were used to, nor something they understood, and so they were naturally suspicious to start with. So long as we explain different relationships and family structures to children, they'll be able to accept them as normal, valid choices, and won't feel threatened or defensive.'*

Top tips

These top tips focus on how to talk to the school about being an LGBT family. This could be when you're choosing a school, meeting a new class teacher or when a concern arises during your child's time at school.

1. **Arrange a time**. Your child's class teacher may meet or visit all new parents as a matter of course, or the school may have regular times when parents can meet with teachers

or governors. You can take these opportunities or set up a separate meeting when there is time to talk without crowds of other parents around.

2. **Explain clearly.** Make sure that, by the end of the meeting, the teacher is clear about who is in your family, and about the language that your child is comfortable using to describe their family. This will vary from family to family. Be clear if there are things that you want the teachers to know but that you don't want shared more widely, or if there is action that you need them to take to address a problem.

3. **Write it down.** This can help get your thoughts clear, and be useful for teachers to refer to later. You could send a follow-up email confirming what you have discussed. If you are talking about a problem, writing down what you want to say first can prevent you missing a crucial point and can also prevent the discussion from getting too heated.

4. **Don't be afraid to ask questions.** You don't have to be Cherry Healey or Jeremy Paxman, but you do need to be happy that you have enough information to make the right decisions for your child. Stonewall's list below gives some starter questions for parents choosing a school.

5. **Listen.** Give the teacher a chance to ask you any questions too. If they are awkward or use the wrong words, it could be because they haven't met any LGBT families before and don't know what to say, rather than because they are hostile.

6. **Offer resources.** Stonewall and Inclusion for All have tons of training, lesson plans, DVDs and reading lists to help schools tackle homophobia and to teach about different families. Your school may already have these – the colourful 'Different Families, Same Love' posters are a giveaway. But if not, you can point the staff in the right direction. Ask if they have books which feature LGBT families – and if not, lend them any that you have at home.

Questions to ask when choosing a school

- Are you a Stonewall School Champion?
- Do you have an anti-bullying policy which specifically mentions homophobic bullying?

- How is the school's stance on homophobic bullying/use of language communicated to pupils?
- What is your procedure for responding to homophobic bullying?
- Are staff given training, as part of their continuous professional development, about different families and ways to make sure that the children of gay parents are supported/included?
- Are you aware of children within the school who have same-sex parents?
- Do you stock books which look at a range of different families?
- How do you include different families such as same-sex families in your curriculum?
- Do you include same-sex relationships as part of sex and relationship education?
- Do you have openly LGBT members of your governing board or staff?
- Do you display posters or other materials around school which celebrate difference, including sexual orientation, in a positive light?

(*Source*: Stonewall)

Special Feature: Cross-cultural parenting

Pride and Joy *focuses on the experiences of LGBT parents in the UK and Ireland – but love knows no borders. As people move between countries for work or study, cross-cultural relationships become increasingly common. So what is it like starting an LGBT family in a country where there's no legal protection for same-sex couples bringing up children, and not much understanding of alternative families? Lil, who is British and lives in Japan with her partner and their one-year-old son, sheds some light on being an expat LGBT parent.*

Lil met her Japanese partner, Kaoru, who was divorced with two older children, while Kaoru was studying in England. After having a civil partnership in the UK, which is not recognised in Japan, they moved to Japan together and Lil started trying to get pregnant.

I was very keen on having children. Kaoru was less enthusiastic as she already had children, was trying to set up her career and was worried about the economic implications. We wanted our child to have Japanese nationality. So we needed to find a Japanese sperm donor who was willing to recognise the child as legally his, even though that would leave a record that he had a child outside of his 'family register', which is like a family tree held at the state's register office. We needed someone responsible enough to be a suitable donor and deal with this, but irresponsible or rebellious enough not to mind if this bothered his family and disrupted the Japanese family register system.

We looked in various places, including on a Japanese Internet site for 'friendship-marriage' aimed at lesbian and gay people who want to marry each other and have a family life together. For some, this is a way to avoid discrimination or to please their parents, others were gay men who couldn't imagine a happy gay family life, so did want a 'genuine' marriage in order to have children. But I wasn't looking to get married; I was already in a partnership with Kaoru!

We also asked a lot of people, and finally after a couple of years found a guy who was perfect for us. He seems to be basically straight in terms of sexual orientation, but hangs out a lot in the queer community. We have recommended him to several other people since, so our son could soon end up with half-siblings.

We have a contract, covering finances, custody and so on, all the specifics, and we got a lawyer to help us write it. It is legally binding, as much as any other private contract, although we don't know how it would be judged if we would, for some reason, have to go through court procedures. But at least it makes all our intentions clear. We won't ask for financial support. Without the contract if I died, the 'father' would be next of kin, but we arranged that first Kaoru and after her my brother would look after our son. This kind of planning about life and death is very puzzling to Japanese people. At first Kaoru also thought it was over the top, but later said that the whole process of talking and thinking about it was useful.

No lawyers here in Japan have any experience in this. We wrote the basic contract and then shared it with them, but they still made mistakes. For example, it wasn't until I was already pregnant that we found out that, for our child to be legally registered by a man, I needed to have a certificate declaring I was single, which they expected the British government to provide. Except of course I wasn't single, we were in a civil partnership. The local city hall registry office had to check with the Japanese Ministry of Justice and Foreign Office about what to do. The British Embassy provided a letter saying such certificates do not exist in the UK. Finally the application was passed after I wrote a declaration that I was 'unmarried'. As Japan doesn't recognise our civil partnership in any other way – I'm treated as single for tax, migration and housing – they couldn't really turn round and change their mind about its status now. This all took three months, during which time I was getting bigger and bigger.

At the clinic where I gave birth and another clinic we checked out, we told them how I got pregnant by home insemination, and two different obstetricians asked, 'Is that possible?' You'd think doctors would know, but they seemed unaware of the physical processes! They were interested though ('You can really do that?'), not disapproving.

When we told Kaoru's parents that I was pregnant, they said, 'Oh no, does that mean we won't see Lil around any more then?' They were bewildered; they thought I was pregnant with someone else's child – which was biologically true! – and was leaving Kaoru. But once they understood, they accepted it. Kaoru's older children are now adults. The oldest got married last year and we were all invited to the wedding – even my parents who were over here from England to see our son. In the formal introductions that take place at Japanese weddings, Kaoru's adult daughter introduced our son as her younger brother and me as her mother's partner. Her husband's family are very respectable and conservative. You could imagine them thinking: 'What? She's who? Who *are* all these foreigners?' But being polite Japanese people, they greeted us as normal. Although our son doesn't know much about it now, it will make a difference to him to see that kind of welcome within the family.

In general, people don't recognise Kaoru as our son's mother until they are told. He looks very Western to them, although he would look slightly Japanese to an English person. They do see a family relationship because of how we communicate with each other, but they can't figure it out. She is that bit older, so often they will think she is his grandma. It's irritating, but at least they recognise something. As our son was born outside the marriage system, and I'm a foreigner, we can choose any surname for him. So we used Kaoru's surname, which helps her role to be recognised.

People who do know don't comment, so I don't know what they think. I'm part of a group of mostly middle-class first-time mums. They've met Kaoru, and they treat her as a woman, but also something like they treat all the husbands. There's a gender divide in Japan, with men working long hours and women often at home. And the same is true with us: I am at home at the moment while Kaoru is working. They like to grumble about their husbands and I sometimes purposefully join in because it normalises it – and of course sometimes I do need to grumble!

We have never made any secret of our relationship. But at the same time, we don't go around saying we are lesbians – we are both bisexuals anyway. Gay people here are not very visible, although recently gay marriage has become topical with a few people having symbolic 'marriages'. Our life is a balancing act between being groundbreaking and being normal enough to be accepted. It's tiring doing that all the time. As a gay person, you can be made to feel like you are representing all gay people. As a foreigner, you're used as a representative for all foreigners. I don't always want to be perceived that way. In the West, there are lots of 'out' role models, so you play less of a representative role. In Japan there are no legal rights or protections for gay couples, there's no institutional awareness, but you can come out and no one is rude to you in public because Japanese people don't do that. You can live here and not fear violence, as sometimes has been the case in the West.

There's no concept of Pride. They do have marches, but these are Rainbow marches, not Pride marches; it's not rights-based. It's more about showing that we are normal people trying to get on with our lives in peace. It makes a difference that Kaoru and I are educated, we have economic means and try to be very reasonable. I think if there was something else noticeable to dislike about us, apart from us being gay, then we would have encountered discrimination. But because we present ourselves in ways we know they'll like – Kaoru is a university professor, I'm a native English-speaker from the West – people have a different attitude.

I've found that you need more time to plan a family in a cross-cultural context. Knowing the law is very difficult in a country where you are essentially illiterate. Being flexible enough to go with the cultural norms is very important. Our son has different parents in different countries – under UK law Kaoru and I are both his parents, but his biological dad is not recognised; and in Japanese law it's his biological dad and me, Kaoru is unrecognised.

As a therapist, I work with international couples, so I understand something about what makes them work and what makes them fall apart. Having a thorough knowledge of each other's cultures beforehand really helps. You might assume it's not very different, but it is. I think LGBT couples are sometimes better off in that respect, they've had to step outside their cultural norms anyway to come out, they've thought more about it and gone through the hurdles sooner, but on the other hand some of the societal supports in place for heterosexual couples are not available to us.

Special Feature:
Relationships under pressure

LGBT families face the same problems as any other families. Parents who identify as lesbian, gay, bi or trans, as well as those who identify as straight, can face divorce, relationship breakdown or can lose contact with their children. It's not all hearts and flowers and rainbow flags. LGBT parents can also face extra pressures, if family members, communities or the legal system fail to recognise or support our families and relationships.

No one finds it easy to share stories of the difficult times, especially when that means acknowledging the part we played ourselves in things going wrong. In particular, we may feel an expectation as LGBT parents to only talk about when things go well, in order to prove that our relationships are valid, to show that we can bring up happy, well-balanced children or to win the approval of wider society.

Yet, it's essential we share the messy, complicated and painful stories too, because they are also part of the experience of being an LGBT parent. We are very grateful to Jon, who is gay and has a grown-up daughter, for being willing to share his experience.

Claiming my experience of fatherhood as 'LGBT parenting' may not be quite accurate. When my daughter was born in 1993 I had not begun to explore my sexual orientation – let alone assumed the identity of a gay man. However, I believe my sexuality has influenced the course of my relationship with my daughter which has led, sadly, to our current estrangement.

I had met her mother a couple of years before my daughter came along when I took up lodgings in her home. She was ten years older than I and had a young son from a previous relationship. I got on well with both of them and we fell into a family relationship which provided mutual support for all of us.

We had not planned the pregnancy and when my daughter was born I was thrust into fatherhood both young and inexperienced. My parents in particular were shocked and angry. Despite these obstacles we attempted to create a loving home for our daughter and, apart from some early health problems, our daughter thrived – becoming a bright, beautiful baby.

As a result of the stress I was experiencing in my new role, I began to struggle in my work and personal life and sought counselling. It was around this time I first considered seriously the possibility of being gay. Though I was able to share something of my doubts with my partner, I was unable – within the context of family and work life, and my own fears – to explore the issue in any depth.

From the middle of 1994, my relationship with my partner began to deteriorate. We argued frequently and I became aware, both as an unmarried father and as a tenant in her house, that I had little support for my role in the family. My relationship with my daughter – though loving – was similarly fragile and unprotected by law. I sought legal advice and tried to obtain parental responsibility – something my ex vehemently opposed.

As I became more desperate, the hostilities increased. Eventually, I moved out of the family home, though still trying to negotiate and maintain contact with the children. I began to suffer from the stress-related illness that led eventually to a 20-year struggle with chronic fatigue syndrome.

When solicitors became involved, the situation was further inflamed. Visits to the children became sporadic amidst the threat of mutual violence between my ex and me. On one occasion we fought bitterly, resulting in my assaulting her.

A legal battle for contact began which was to drag on for several years. Unwilling to abandon my daughter, I fought to maintain our relationship but this antagonised my ex who wanted me to have nothing more to do with the family. Eventually, she alleged that I had sexually abused my daughter and while these claims were dismissed in court, an image of me as a sexually unstable, violent character was established. I believe that the stereotype of the homosexual as a potential child abuser was also in the background.

Finally, the judge ordered that my daughter and I should have indirect contact with items such as birthday cards and gifts passed through my ex's solicitor. Over the next fifteen years or so I communicated with my daughter only by sending gifts at Christmas and at Jewish New Year. For many years, I received no acknowledgment, but later on she sent me occasional emails thanking me and telling me something about her life. I never received a photo however, and have neither seen nor heard her since she was two years old. She is now 24.

In 2014, I decided that I was no longer prepared to maintain a relationship mediated through a solicitor. Having explained my reasons to my daughter and encouraged her – when the time was right – to contact me as an independent adult, I terminated contact. To date, I have not heard from her, but I trust that she will approach me when she chooses.

Over the duration of our contact, I explained a little of my life, and of the difficulties which led to our separation, to my daughter. I have never hidden my sexuality from her. In any case, my work as a musician and author has involved putting some of my private life in the public domain.

As I have become more accepting of myself as a gay man, I have come to understand and have compassion for the painful events which affected our family so many years ago. I now have many LGBT friends, including a number of gay men who also have adult children. Many of them have maintained relationships with their children, sometimes very close ones. Although that has not been my experience, I have never for a moment regretted being a father. Nor have I ever doubted that one day my daughter will want to know me again, and that I shall be able to stand proudly before her as a gay man embracing his wonderful daughter.

Part Three

Creating new forms of family

11

BIOLOGY ISN'T DESTINY

Many LGBT families include parents who are not genetically related to their children, and siblings who have no biological connection to each other. There may be biological 'parents' who don't take on a parental role, and biological relatives who remain unknown. This chapter looks at the significance of genetic connections or the lack of them within families; explores how people decide whether or not to become biological parents; and finds out how non-biological parents define and defend their roles.

What makes a parent? Is it genetics – the mysterious strands of DNA weaving patterns through the generations? Or is it proximity – being there for sleepless nights and nappy changes, for bar mitzvahs and graduation ceremonies? Or is it all in the name – ensuring that your children know you as their mum or dad? Genetics, proximity and naming. Each of these is part of what it means to be a parent. But how much do they matter? This is an emotive issue, about which views are held strongly and feelings can be hard to rationalise or explain.

Does biology matter? Adoptive parents speak out

Adoptive parents have children who are biologically unrelated to themselves. During months of adoption preparation, they have had to reflect on their choice to adopt and explore its implications. These parents and their children create families through legal decree, and through shared experiences, rather than shared DNA. Few of those who we spoke to would have it any other way.

'*I don't know what it's like to have a biological child*,' reflects Janice, who has two adopted daughters. '*But when I tuck my two up in bed and gaze at them as they sleep, I feel an awesome amount of love. Biology seems irrelevant.*' This doesn't mean that Janice and her ex-partner hide the fact that their children are not genetically related to them. '*We are very open with them about their adoptions and birth families,*' she continues. '*But we share our values, interests and expressions and I think that all contributes to us becoming a family. We are parents. That means the same thing no matter how you get there.*'

'*I don't think it matters, not being blood related,*' agrees Bronwen, who adopted her daughter at nine years old. '*She has picked up my mannerisms, people say she looks like me and she says things I say! Her friends don't believe her if she tells them she's adopted.*' Bronwen thinks there *are* differences in the way you parent an adopted child, even if there is no difference in how much you love them. '*Loving an adopted child, I'm guessing, is different to bringing up a birth child, especially if you have missed out on the early years,*' she considers. '*Children who are late-adopted usually have very difficult backgrounds and may find it hard to form relationships. This means I have to be a different type of parent. I am not adopted, and I parent my daughter therapeutically, a very different way from how I was parented myself.*'

Andrew and his partner adopted their son when he was very young. Unlike Bronwen's daughter, he will have little conscious memory of life before he came to live with his two dads. '*Over the 14 months he has been with us, we have seen a massive change in his personality, his speech, his learning – everything!*' says Andrew. '*We learnt a lot about nature and nurture in our pre-adoption training; all we learnt then is coming to life now! Inevitably, our son will have his own personality and deal with things differently to us. We see him copy a lot of things we are doing and he learns a lot from those around him too. In this respect, it doesn't matter that we don't have a genetic relationship with him. He can be "moulded" by us, but he will be whoever he is meant to be.*'

Parents who know little about their child's genetic heritage, whether because their child is adopted or because their child was conceived through anonymous egg or sperm donation, may be anxious that difficulties or surprises might lie in store as their child grows up. Andrew and his partner recognise that this could be the case with their son, but are not unduly worried. *'Before we adopted our son social workers gave us an idea of the potential issues this little boy could face as he grew up,'* explains Andrew. *'But, who knows what will be in five, ten or 15 years' time? No one knows this, even with their biological children. All we knew was that this little boy would get all the love, support and nurture he needed from two very loving and caring daddies.'*

For many LGBT couples considering adoption, this path is their first choice, sometimes in part because it puts both parents-to-be on an equal footing: neither parent will be assumed to have a deeper bond than the other based on genetic connection. This was the case for Janice and her partner at the time. *'One of us could have conceived,'* she says. *'But I wanted us to have an equal relationship with the children. There are beautiful kids out there who needed stability and love. For us, this was the best decision ever.'*

'But who's the real father?':
When one parent is bio, and one is not

At present, same-sex couples cannot both be genetic parents of a child. Medical technology can do a lot – it can even enable one partner in a lesbian couple to donate eggs to her partner, so that one is the genetic mother and the other is the birth mother – but it can't yet knit the genetic material of two men or two women together to form a new person. There are some couples who use both donor eggs and donor sperm, meaning that neither partner has a genetic relationship to their children.

Does any of this matter? Who cares who's biologically related to whom? In a society where many children are brought up by step-parents or adoptive parents or, whether they know it or not, were conceived using donated sperm or eggs as part of fertility treatment, or even on a one-night stand, what's all the fuss about?

Yet it does matter. Although not in a 'who is the *real* parent?' sort of way. Even if in your own mind biological relatedness genuinely doesn't matter, it is something that others seem to be endlessly curious about. Whether you like it or not, the questions will come, as Bryony knows from experience.

'Biology doesn't matter at all to me, but it clearly matters to

other people,' says Bryony, who was brought up from the age of five by her mum and her mum's partner, Sue. '*I've been asked all sorts, from "do you love Sue as much as your mum?" to "you must love your mum most because you don't live with your dad and Sue isn't even related to you". I've been told that my family from Sue's side aren't my "real family", and it's implied that I can't really be that close to them.*'

Bryony has a simple response: '*I brush these things off as ridiculous. Within the family, we've always maintained that the lack of a biological link between Sue and me is irrelevant, as we lived together for so long and she has raised me. I am much closer to some of Sue's family than I am to some of my mum or dad's families. Yet when I explain this to people, it's hard to really get through to them. Even close friends have said things without thinking, like explaining why they want to have their "own children". I think that the desire for biological ties is incredibly strong, and that it is a natural and hormonal force. However, I firmly believe that the love between non-biologically related people can be just as strong.*'

Sue's family have quietly but deliberately shown Bryony that she is part of their family too. Their words and actions have been enormously important to Bryony. '*Sue's sister told me one day that she considered me her niece and that she loved me very much and I was never to think otherwise. Before he died, Sue's dad told me the same thing. Both times, I was surprised. I didn't feel that these things needed to be said, but I was deeply touched that they had said them,*' she remembers. The family knew that other people might cast doubt on their relationships, and wanted Bryony to know how significant they were. She continues, '*Over the years, I think every person in that family has said the same thing to me! I'm very lucky as I know that not all families are so accepting.*'

Jess, now in her 20s, was conceived using an anonymous sperm donor, brought up by her two mums, and has one sister who was conceived with sperm from a different donor. Like Bryony, she often has to justify the close relationship she has with non-biological relatives. '*I have often been asked if I love my biological mother more than my non-biological mother or if I don't get on with my sister because she's only my "half"-sister,*' says Jess. '*I have never felt any of these things. My mums are both my parents and my sister is my sister,*' she adds firmly. '*Having a biological link to me doesn't matter at all. Physically, I look a lot like my biological mum, but character-wise I am a perfect match with both of my parents.*'

For Jess, it's social and legal status, not genetic inheritance, that matters. Having a legal connection to her non-biological mum would have helped her answer some of the questions she faced as a child. She continues, '*I'm so glad that the law has changed now and both LGBT parents can be on the birth certificate. It was different when I was conceived. I am not legally connected to my non-biological mum in any way. I think this has had a negative effect on her and has sometimes made it difficult to explain her relationship to me and my sister.*'

Han, who also has two mums, recognises that '*every time it comes up that I have lesbian parents I get a lot of questions, like whether I'm adopted or do I know my sperm donor. They're never insulting. I think people are just curious and so I answer them honestly.*'

So is honesty the best policy? To try to minimise the differences between non-biological and biological parents, some couples refuse to reveal who is biologically related to whom, while others try to pre-empt questions by providing information up front. Both strategies can end up making biology seem a bigger issue than it really is, a problem that lesbian mum Heather has recently been reflecting on. '*I attended a workshop not long ago where I had to introduce my family,*' she says. '*I did what I always do – I said that I was one of a two-mum family and we had two children; I had the first one and my partner had the second, but they have the same donor father. One of the participants asked me at the break why I felt the need to differentiate between the two children.*'

'*I was thrown when I was asked this question. My description was an automatic response to the questions which often follow – "Who had who?" "Are they adopted?" "Who's the daddy?" I thought that if I could answer all of these in one or two sentences then that would stop any further questions. But I am glad to have been challenged because now I won't be describing us in that way again – I will simply say, "I am one of a two-mum*' *family and we have two children."*

Felix and Evan, who started their family via surrogacy, were so keen that their friends and family would see them as equal parents that they decided not to reveal which of them was their son's biological father. It's a decision which now they think might have made people more obsessed about biological connection, rather than less. *'Everyone tried to guess and wanted to talk about it,'* remembers Evan. *'We don't look that different from each other: our son looks like us both, so it could have been either of us. A friend asked us, "Come on, tell us, who's the real father?" We said: "That's exactly the point." He felt awful about it. We didn't want to make a big deal of it, but actually that made it a bigger issue.'*

Felix agrees: *'If we could do it again, I'd be much more open.'* Now that all the family do know, it hasn't made any difference to their relationships; both sets of doting grandparents still dote as much as ever. But their two-year-old son, despite knowing about the surrogate and the egg donor who helped make him, doesn't yet know – and hasn't yet asked – which of his dads is his biological dad. *'I'm less bothered about telling him early because he doesn't understand it, even if for us it makes the story complete,'* continues Felix. *'He doesn't have to understand at two years old that one of his dads is a more fundamental part of him than the other.'*

To bio or to non-bio, that is the question

If you're in a same-sex couple and only one of you can be the biological parent, how do you choose who it's going to be? Well, it could be the one who...

...is keenest on/less freaked out by the whole baby plan

...cares most about having a genetic link to the child

...most wants their nationality or ethnic identity to be passed on

...has the job with the most generous maternity/paternity leave

...doesn't like their job and fancies a few months at home

...wins at a game of 'scissors, paper, stone' or a coin toss

...is younger/more fertile

...most wants to experience pregnancy and birth

The experience of pregnancy, birth and family life can change your perspective, as well as external factors like job changes or family support. It's important to be ready to revisit decisions that made sense at the time, in the light of how you feel later. Jessica and her partner planned to take turns to be the biological mother, but it was clear who was going to have the first go. *'It was very straightforward to decide,'* says Jessica. *'It was always in my view of life that I would be pregnant, and of course I was a whole year older at 31! Getting pregnant was something I felt confident about, although we always said we'd have one each.'*

That wasn't how it turned out. *'Parenting teaches you that you can have a plan, but things evolve and your family changes,'* continues Jessica. *'Early on, we thought it was important that we both had the chance to get pregnant, but I was happy to go through it again and my partner didn't mind. She's said that watching your partner give birth is the most awesome, mind-blowing experience. Who gave birth is of secondary importance to us, the birth bit soon passes. We are both completely their parents.'*

It's a personal decision. For some, like Jessica and her partner, it will fall into place. For others, it will be more complicated. Bodies and biology are capricious, and there's no guarantee that carefully devised plans will work. Kim and her partner gave birth to one of their children each, although that was not their original plan. *'I wanted to have a biological child and to experience pregnancy, whereas my partner didn't,'* explains Kim. *'Therefore we planned for me to try to conceive a child, and hopefully more in the future.'* So far, so good. Kim successfully conceived and gave birth to a healthy baby, but spent much of her pregnancy in hospital with severe vomiting. Her extremely difficult pregnancy meant that they had to revise their plans, as another pregnancy like the first would be even harder for them to manage while caring for a toddler. Something else changed too. *'My partner started to have a desire to become pregnant,'* says Kim. *'I think it was partly due to experiencing my pregnancy, although I'm not sure why it didn't put her off, and also due to the tragic suicide of her father when our son was just a few weeks old.'*

However, this wasn't easy for Kim to accept: '*Most people did, and still do, rightly point out how lucky we are that we can both carry a child. People often joke about how they wish their husband or male partner could have carried their child. However, it's not as simple as that. These comments were often unhelpful, due to my own mixed emotions and my longing to carry another child and experience a healthy pregnancy. As I had reduced to part-time hours after our son was born, this change of roles impacted on us financially too.*'

When Hannah and her partner first talked about having children they knew one thing: '*I wanted to be pregnant and my wife didn't,*' says Hannah. Even so, they regretted not both being able to have a biological connection to their child. Then Hannah's partner came up with an idea: '*She couldn't inseminate me, but she could give me her eggs. We had no idea if this was possible because we didn't know much about assisted reproduction, only knew lesbian parents online and had only seen the traditional turkey baster method in the films.*' So Hannah started emailing fertility clinics to find out more. '*We were so excited when we received a few replies to say that this was possible. It was the perfect answer for us: I would be the birth mother and my wife the biological mother. I feel really proud of the fact that our daughter is biologically my wife's and smile to myself when people comment on how much she looks like me, assuming that I'm her biological mother.*'

While it's often the partner who sees herself as being 'more maternal' who opts to be the biological mum, this was not the case for Tricia and her partner. '*Initially, we agreed I would carry the baby, since my partner saw herself in a more "dad" role. But we ended up switching,*' Tricia explains. '*Although my partner feels less "motherly" (her words) and has less experience with children, it became apparent that she felt more strongly about a genetic link to the baby (and thus, perhaps passing on her identity as a Latina) while I wasn't worried about being genetically related.*' Tricia now feels this arrangement will make it easier for them both to play full and confident parenting roles: '*I am very into the idea of parenting and I think not being the biological parent gives me more impetus to get involved.*'

Another way of redressing the balance is for the non-biological parent to become the main caregiver. But this can be practically and financially hard for lesbian couples, when the first six months of maternity leave is granted to the birth mother only. The good news is that recent legal changes mean that the second six months of leave can be taken by either parent, which gives a chance to even things up. For gay male couples using surrogacy to have a child, there can be more flexibility in who takes leave, since a change in the law in 2015 created a statutory obligation for employers to grant leave.

Defining your role as a non-bio parent

When Felix and Evan started thinking about parenthood, it was not clear who would be the biological dad. '*At the time we assumed we'd get a bunch of eggs and fertilise half each and implant those which worked best,*' says Felix. Nice idea – but it didn't work out like that. '*There weren't enough eggs to do half each, so we had to pick who it would be. We were given five minutes to decide, so we tossed a coin. That was it. We were hoping science would make the decision, but actually it was a ten pence piece.*'

The couple decided that the non-bio dad would stay at home with their son in the first few months. '*It kind of balances it out,*' he explains. '*There's a risk for the non-biological parent otherwise that the child is not perceived as your own, and every time he cried I put it down to the fact I wasn't his biological dad. It was ridiculous.*'

Ridiculous, maybe. But hardly unusual. As a non-bio parent, you probably planned the pregnancy together with your partner, witnessed the birth and got to know your baby from their first cry and first cuddle. Yet despite this early bonding, non-bio mums and dads can be secretly worried they won't feel like a 'proper parent' or be recognised as such because they don't have a genetic connection to their children. '*It is often insinuated that we should or do have closer bonds with our own birth child,*' says Kim, who gave birth to one of her children and not to the other. '*But I bonded a lot quicker with my (non-birth) daughter than I did my (birth) son.*' While some parents do feel a closer connection, at least at first, to a biological child than a non-biological one, Kim's experience contradicts the assumption that genetic bonds are necessarily the strongest.

Hannah and her partner, who chose egg-sharing IVF to start their family, insist that the biggest lesson they've learnt on their journey to parenthood is 'that it is unconditional love that makes family', rather than how a child is conceived or whether or not there is a biological link between parent and child. But in the back of their minds, they still feel that 'it is easier for other people to accept us both as our daughter's mums, because of the roles we both played in her birth. While I grew her in my womb, and I gave birth to her and breastfed her, my wife has the biological connection.'

The tricky business of working out your role as a non-bio mum starts during your partner's pregnancy or even earlier. Non-bio mum Sally's feelings are recognisable, not only to other non-bio mums, but also to dads-to-be in straight relationships. 'One of the challenges of being the partner of a pregnant woman is finding your role,' she says. 'My partner gets to be part of this secret society of women who give each other knowing looks, roll their eyes in unison and shake their heads over things such as pelvic floors and pregnancy pillows. The first question, understandably, that anyone asks me is how my partner is. There is an assumption that I am fine, making cups of tea and soaking up the stress. I don't have an automatic role. I'm not a "dad" but I'm not a "mum" in the traditional sense either. It's quite nice, to be left to find my own way and do it the way that feels right. But sometimes, it is hard to work out what I should be doing. I hope that my partner feels supported by me, and I am fortunate that when I have a "parental wobble" she is there and willing to listen.'

It doesn't get more straightforward after the birth. 'It's taken me a few years to settle into my role as a non-biological mum and work out what it is,' says Mich, whose daughter is now eight years old. 'It's obvious what's expected of a father. There are plenty of gender stereotypes about how a dad should be. There wasn't really anything to go on with my role; consequently, I found myself taking on a bit of a fatherly role. Talking to heterosexual friends, my female friends would say, "Yes, my husband feels like that," about things I was feeling. I did feel a little bit pushed out of the bonding between the baby and my partner through breastfeeding. It was difficult feeling this amid the joy of having a new child.' Although the 'dad' role was a partial fit for Mich, she had to develop her own role in the absence of role models. 'The three of us just made up the role for ourselves: me reacting to what my partner and the baby needed from me,' she explains.

'I think it's harder to be a woman supporting your partner to breastfeed, than it is for a man,' says Marie, who gave birth to their son. 'This was one area where I had not expected biology to make such a difference in our parenting, but it did. We got off to such a rocky start with breastfeeding that we needed to focus our energy on making breastfeeding work. Therefore, it couldn't be the case that Beth gave him an occasional bottle. This meant that, at first, our son bonded very closely with me.'

Babies are not renowned for their tact. Their main focus is getting their basic needs met – and if you haven't got milk on tap at the exact moment they want it, they're not interested. Even if you know rationally that you are a good and loving parent without having a biological link to your child or being able to breastfeed them, no one is thinking totally rationally after nights of broken sleep and heightened emotions, especially when you're holding a screaming, purple-faced baby demanding to be fed. Although a few non-bio mums have a go at breastfeeding alongside the baby's biological mum, using breast pumps and medication to stimulate milk production, this is still rare.

'He would want to be with Marie, he would push me away,' continues Beth. 'Sometimes he'd go for my boobs and I'd make a joke of it.' But it passed. 'When Marie went away with work for a week, he'd cuddle up to me to go to sleep. He wouldn't have done that before.'

She looks just like you

Even when people know which of you is the biological mum and which isn't, it's still easy for them to forget. Lesbian couple Amy and Pally were surprised by a comment that came only seconds after their son was born. 'The midwives at the hospital fully involved both of us,' says bio-mum Amy. 'We had a water *birth and Pally got in the tub with me. The funniest thing was when I gave birth to our son, the midwife commented, "Ooh, hasn't he got Pally's eyes!"*

Nicholas also found that hospital staff were keen to include him in all aspects of the pregnancy and birth, even those which weren't completely relevant to him as a non-bio dad. *'All the medical staff were very supportive and excited for us, while of course prioritising our surrogate's health and the health of the baby,'* he remembers. *'They even asked me for my medical history and wrote it all down! It could be a different story elsewhere, but we had beautiful care. We were all included.'*

Non-bio mum Beth went back to work shortly after her partner gave birth to their son, sparking confusion among her colleagues. *'A colleague I didn't know very well said to me, "You've just had a baby, haven't you? You're back at work already, what are you – superwoman?" and then bustled off again before I could explain,'* Beth remembers. *'Not long after that, I had a casual conversation with a different colleague about putting on weight. She said, "Oh, well, you have just had a baby, haven't you?" I didn't have the heart to say that I hadn't put on weight because I'd given birth, instead we were both finding new parenthood so exhausting that I was eating lots of chocolate!'*

For the most part, people see what they want to see. They make assumptions and fit the pieces together in the way that seems to make most sense. If people expect you to be the biological parent or assume that your child will look like you, then that's what they'll see. But the comment 'she looks just like you' or 'he's got your eyes' addressed to a non-bio mum or dad by well-meaning strangers or friends can elicit different reactions, from amusement to delight, annoyance to confusion.

Although they can be funny, 'she looks like you' comments can suggest that physical resemblance is the defining feature of parenthood. *'Lots of people, who know I'm not the biological mother, say, "Oh, he looks so like you,"'* continues Beth. *'It's meant in a nice way, but it wouldn't matter if I didn't look like him at all, he's still my son.'*

That's how Jenny feels too. Neither she nor her partner, Lucy, has a genetic link to their children as they used an egg donor to get pregnant. *'It makes it a bit fairer somehow, that they are not* biologically related to either of us,' says Jenny. 'But they spent nine months in Lucy's womb, that must make a difference, and she was off work for a year with each of them.' Because Lucy was the birth mother, those who don't know otherwise assume that she does have a genetic connection. That, and the hair. 'My children don't look like me at all,' says Jenny. 'They do look like Lucy, especially our daughter who has hair like hers, so you wouldn't know. People often say to Lucy, "She looks just like you" or "Her hair's just like yours". I never get that. It can be hard to feel that people don't see the connection between you and your children. I'm definitely their mum, one of their mums, but if they're not biologically related to you it's very difficult to see yourself in them. Maybe it's a good thing, like if they've got a bad temper and you've got a bad temper, you can't just say, "Oh, they've inherited it from me." It makes them more their own person.'

When Sally's daughter was very young, a news story broke about children being removed from their Roma parents. The children had been taken by police, who assumed they had been kidnapped because they did not look like their parents. 'From what I gathered, a child was taken by the authorities because she was blonde and not connected to her parents by DNA,' says Sally, explaining how her outrage at this news story made her stop and think about what being a non-biological parent meant to her. 'On that basis, in a few years' time I should expect police to come sniffing around me and my daughter. She will almost certainly have different colouring to me and definitely has no DNA connection to me. That doesn't make her any less my daughter. I helped bring her into the world, change her nappies, cuddle her, care for her and fear for the future for her, as most parents do. Of course, I am not Roma, and therein lies my safety.' Sally recognises the other factors at play here, in particular the racism surrounding Roma people. But it also reinforced her beliefs about how insignificant biology, or even resemblance, can be in defining who is or isn't a parent.

'The biological stuff means very little to me now,' she continues. 'I started blogging when my partner was pregnant to deal with the fallout of not being biologically linked to my child. It felt like a big deal then. But now, months on, I feel without question I am this child's mama. The donor was just that, a *donor. And while I am grateful for what he did, it is me who has supported my partner through the pregnancy, sat by her side in the birthing suite, and who is bringing up our daughter. In my view parenting has bugger all to do with DNA or ethnicity, and everything to do with love and responsibility.'*

It's in the genes

For every non-biological parent, there will be a biological parent or donor: someone somewhere whose sperm or egg helped create the child. In the UK, laws surrounding donor anonymity changed in 2005 to allow children conceived via sperm and egg donation to contact the donor when they reach adulthood. It's too early to tell how this will turn out. We don't know how many people will want to seek out the donor. But, if 25-year-old Jess's experience is anything to go by, there will be many for whom this is only of passing interest.

'Growing up without a father never felt like having a gap to fill,' says Jess. *'As far as I was concerned, I had two loving parents who wanted me and cared for me – why should having a male parent be any different, or even desirous? As he was an anonymous donor, I don't have the option to find out any details about him. However, this has never bothered me. I'm not interested in finding out who my donor was, nor forming any relationship with him.'*

Other children of LGBT parents are more curious about their genetic identity. Parents who've used donor sperm or eggs to conceive can be curious too. Jim is a transman and he and his wife, Katie, used donor sperm at a clinic to conceive their two sons. They know very little about the donor or, consequently, about that part of their children's genetic heritage. But they do wonder sometimes about what he is like. *'Everything we know about this man is written on one piece of paper. Apart from of course what we know through the boys,'* says Katie. *'I think I would recognise his hands if I saw them, and I suspect he's quite artistic. Just occasionally I look at random men on the train and wonder...'*

The recent 'donor release' laws have prompted parents to think carefully about when and how they share what they know about their donors with their children. This includes parents whose children were born before the change in the law. 'The boys have no contact with the donor, and no legal right to have any contact,' explains Katie. 'The law changed after our elder son was born, but we wanted them to have the same biological father if possible, and the change didn't apply retrospectively to existing donors. We have talked to them about their donor and we've tried to paint him in a positive light. I am massively grateful to him. Soon we'll let them read the little information we have about him, and if they want to try to find him when they are older, we'll support them.'

For many people, there is a fascination about genetic heritage which is hard to shake; a desire to know where they come from, in order to know who they are now. Apart from the practical advantages of having more than two parents, this is one of the reasons that some lesbians want a co-parent or sperm donor whom they know and whom their children can get to know. At a basic level, it means the child's background and medical history are less of a mystery. At a deeper level, they hope that this bond will enhance their child's life and help them to form their own identity.

David, who donated sperm to a lesbian couple, has always played a role in his daughter's life, seeing her every six weeks or so. He has a close friendship with her two mums, which has grown over the years. 'We don't use the word "co-parents". All I've been is a steady presence in the background,' he says. 'We've been on holiday together or away for the weekend, and I know they talk about me when I'm not there.' But David believes it's not just the time he's spent with his daughter that has helped shaped who she is – genes come into it somehow too. 'I'm sure a few things from me do rub off. I believe that genetics, nature as much as nurture, makes a difference,' he explains. 'I notice it with my daughter. My friends have too. I've seen some definite similarities to me, which she can't simply have picked up from me. Lots of her personality mirrors mine.'

Jacob had a similar kind of relationship with his biological father when he was growing up. His father didn't live with Jacob or have a parenting role, although they were always very close; rather, Jacob was brought up by his lesbian mum. Yet, Jacob has noticed many similarities between himself and his father. 'I find it interesting how uncannily similar I am to my *father, despite him not having raised me,' ponders Jacob. 'We have similar interests and outlooks on life, have faced similar issues in our personal lives, and share lots of artistic interests. People also say we sound similar on the phone and have similar personalities. I believe that individuals are not biologically predetermined, rather it is a set of outside influences that configure people differently. My similarity to my father seems to go against this somewhat, so it's fascinating for me to consider this when assessing my beliefs around social constructivism.'*

Even Jess, who was brought up by her two mums and clearly has no interest in finding her biological father, feels that genetic links are significant. *'I don't have an interest in finding out who my donor was, nor forming any relationship with him,'* she says firmly, *'but I have signed up to various donor child sites, in order to search for biological siblings.'*

Brotherly – and sisterly – love

Not everyone craves a full house or, whether for practical or emotional reasons, has more than one child. But for many first-time parents, once they've realised they can cope with the sleepless nights and sticky fingers, doing it all over again seems the natural next step. There are many reasons to want more than one child which have nothing to do with being in an LGBT family. You might have memories of playing and fighting, sharing and scrapping with your own siblings and want to recreate that closeness for your own children. Or you might remember being an only child and wondering what it would be like to have a sibling. Yet there are reasons, both social and biological, why LGBT parents in particular can seek to have more than one child.

The social stuff first. All parents are odd and embarrassing at times, whatever the family set-up. And LGBT families, let's face it, are still a little bit unusual. Having two or more children means that they can discuss their weird family together. They will definitely know at least one other person in an LGBT family – even if it's just their own brother or sister!

Genetics come into play too. Having a second child can give both partners in a same-sex couple the opportunity to pass on their genes. If the same donor is used, then the siblings have a genetic connection to each other as well. Jenny and her partner had always hoped to have two children, but struggled to get pregnant with their first. They eventually conceived with donor sperm and eggs, so neither of them had a genetic connection to their son. '*We wanted a second child, but we also wanted our son to have someone he knew he was biologically related to,*' explains Jenny. '*We had some sperm remaining and the clinic asked the woman who donated the eggs the first time whether she'd be happy to donate again. We were really lucky that she was.*'

Some families will include siblings who are genetic half-siblings; for example, a lesbian couple might take turns in getting pregnant, but use the same donor sperm. In other families, there may be siblings who have no biological relationship to each other at all, like Rajo and Varinder's two children. Rajo and Varinder were pregnant at the same time and the children were born only ten days apart. They've probably spent more time with each other growing up than anyone else. It's hardly surprising how close they are. '*The children act like twins,*' says Rajo. '*People assume that they are twins. They are somehow able to communicate, not always speaking but still aware of what the other needs or is doing. People think it would have been logical to have the same donor, but we didn't. They are not biologically related but are still 100% sister and brother. They are similar in how they look and behave, I suppose because they are raised within the same family.*'

Top tips

This chapter's top tips focus on how to negotiate being a non-biological parent.

1. **Prepare your response** People will ask you, your partner and your family about what it's like being a non-bio parent. The questions may be well-meaning and come out of genuine interest, but can be tiring to keep on answering. It's best to be clear in your own mind which questions you will and will not answer. When someone asks whether you are a biological parent, you may be happy to tell them – but you don't have to be. It's no one's business but your own.

2. **Accentuate the positive.** Perhaps being a biological parent was never part of your life plan, or perhaps it was something

you desperately wanted but was not to be. Regardless of whether you chose your role or not, you can still choose to be the best parent you can be. You can define your own role in relation to what your child needs from *you*. You can share your interests, tastes and experiences with your child, responding to them as they look to you and learn from you. You can look into adjusting your working pattern to spend as much of those crucial early months as possible getting to know your child and allowing them to get to know you. This may mean, if you are not out at work, either as LGBT or as a parent, that you have to take the plunge and come out. Becoming a parent is something which is too important to hide.

3. **Go undercover.** Here's the secret. Most of the time people can't tell or don't care if you're a biological parent. So why waste time worrying? During pregnancy, and to a lesser extent during the first year, it's more obvious. But after that, it's anyone's guess.

4. **Make it legal.** Since 2008, both partners in a civil partnership go on the birth certificate as parents. This shows the commitment of both parents to bringing up their child and makes the role of the non-bio parent official. There are other ways to make a public declaration of your commitment to each other as a family, such as using a shared surname or holding a naming ceremony surrounded by friends and family.

5. **Preference often passes.** There may be times in those early, exhausting, anxious weeks when you worry whether you will be able to bond successfully with your child. If this becomes a problem, there are things you can do, such as ensuring you and your child get one-to-one time together. But, above all, you can hold onto the fact that – like teething and sleepless nights – this will pass. Family relationships change and develop as children get older. Each child – and parent for that matter – has their own distinct character and interests. Each child is their own complex mix of nature and nurture. In any family, no parent/child relationship is identical, and that uniqueness in itself should be a great source of pride and joy.

12

THE GENDER AGENDA

This chapter covers how, as LGBT families, we can choose to accept, question or resist traditional gender roles; how we deal with questions about the presence or absence of male or female role models; and how the experience of growing up with LGBT parents can influence our children's attitudes to gender.

One of the greatest fears about lesbian, gay, bi or trans people bringing up children, still expressed by opponents of LGBT families, is that it will spread gender confusion. They worry that children who grow up in LGBT families will be confused about their gender identity or turn out to be lesbian, gay, bisexual or trans themselves.

Even if this were necessarily the case, is having children who are able to question gender roles and find their own path *really* a bad thing? Is bringing up children to be comfortable with their own sexuality *really* a danger? Both seem to be pretty good parenting outcomes, rather than cause for concern. Some LGBT parents have children who go on to identify as LGBT themselves, some have children who identify as straight, and some have both. No different from straight parents.

Lesbian mother Daisy wasn't shocked when her daughter came out, quite the reverse. '*One of the four children I brought up is gay and now has her own children by insemination,*' she explains. '*I can't remember her coming out. When she was 19 she was living with another woman. It wasn't surprising.*'

Despite having two lesbian mums and being brought up in a gay-affirming family, Jess took time to come to terms with being gay herself. '*I had been bullied by a girl at school who said that I "must be a lesbian" because my parents were. I didn't want to prove her right,*' she says. '*I battled with my feelings alone until I was 15 when I told my parents that I thought I might fancy girls. My biological mum was shocked. She had failed to notice my lack of interest in make-up and dolls and assumed that I would grow up to identify as straight. I think a small part of her hoped that I would, just so that she could show that two gay women could raise a straight child. However, my sister has a boyfriend and completely identifies as straight. My non-biological mum wasn't so shocked. She had always known that I could have turned out either way.*

As an active 'Yes' campaigner in the 2015 Irish marriage equality referendum, adoptive dad Dónal encountered the belief that same-sex couples are ill-equipped to bring up children. *'Many of the anti-Marriage Equality campaigners focused on children, rather than admit that they find gay sex to be icky and believe it to be sinful. There was lots of discussion about purposefully depriving children of a mother or father,'* he explains. *'This was hard on our boys. Both were teased in school and we had to spend a lot of time supporting them and reminding them that we didn't remove them from their mother. They were removed because she could not protect them. I find it hard to forgive the "No" campaigners for the stress they caused to our kids and the kids of all LGBT-headed families in Ireland.'*

Legally, much of the shift has already happened: same-sex couples can adopt and foster jointly, and fertility clinics treating lesbians take into account a child's need for 'supportive parenting' rather than their need for a father. But, regardless of the legal situation, and however much we challenge gender roles in our own lives or seek to ensure our children have the same opportunities whatever their gender identity, we encounter gender stereotypes every day at school, in the media and among our friends.

The 70s, 80s and early 90s

Attitudes to gender among LGBT communities, as well as among wider society, have changed over time. LGBT parents in the 70s, 80s and early 90s were legally vulnerable and socially marginalised, and courts generally ruled that LGBT people were unfit to raise their children. LGBT parents often had to hide, or to fight to be accepted as legitimate parents. *'My mothers decided to have children in 1990, when LGBT parenting was rarely heard of,* reflects Jess. *'I have always thought that they were so brave, having children when they did.'*

Jackie became a parent in the early 1990s. *'When I met my partner, she already had a child and was keen to meet someone who wanted to create a family,'* she says. Despite their commitment to each other and to parenting, they had different views about the importance of involving a father in a child's life. *'She had got pregnant through an anonymous donor exchange,'* continues Jackie. *'There was a third party involved and she never knew who the father was. Because of her desperation not to know, she inseminated with sperm from two anonymous donors in the same month. But I didn't want to do it like that.'* So Jackie asked her friend Paul to be a known donor – a decision she's never regretted – and had her son Jacob at the age of 39.

'Jacob calls Paul by his first name, not "Dad", because he's never been a dad,' says Jackie, explaining the kind of relationship they have. *'He's never been involved at all in bringing Jacob up. But I've ensured that, since Jacob was a baby, they've had contact. He came to all Jacob's birthday parties, to his bar mitzvah, to his graduation, to everything.'*

'Starting out now is so different,' she reflects. *'But I'd still say, make sure your children have a known father. I know we're in the 21st century now, but I'd still say it. It's not because I think a man has to be in a child's life, it's just because I think that they deserve to know who their father is. I might be shot down, but I do believe that.'*

Jacob's understanding of gender roles has also been shaped by growing up in a single-parent family for as long as he could remember. Jackie's partner died when he was young, and until his teens, his mum wasn't out as a lesbian. It was her identity as a single parent, rather than her sexual orientation, that was obvious. *'I think my family structure intrinsically challenges gender roles,'* he says. *'My mother had to fulfil the roles typically assigned to two differently gendered parents in a heterosexual relationship. The fact that this was the first thing I knew makes it difficult to understand the arguments of people advocating traditional family make-ups. I've simply never experienced one and don't feel like anything was lacking in mine. LGBT families can be just as great and just as fucked up as any other family.'*

Lesbians having children at that time often saw their feminism as an intrinsic part of their lesbian identity. Some lesbians positioned themselves as separatists, believing that patriarchy was the root of women's oppression. In order for women to be empowered and free, they sought women-only spaces where men were not allowed: '*I hope this doesn't happen any more, but 25 years ago lesbians were saying that they didn't want boys. I found that so obnoxious,*' remembers Jackie. '*But when my son was born, I had a sense of relief that he was a boy. I wondered if I would be able to bring up a girl to be as feminine as she might need or want to be. So when I had a boy, I thought, Phew, I'm going to find this easier. But he was not a conventional boy! I am more of a stereotypical tomboy – the dyke kind of stuff – and my boy, whom I wanted to teach to play football, was not interested.*'

Bringing up their four children in the 1970s, feminism was at the centre of Daisy and her partner's understanding of family. '*We were both feminists, that informs the kind of lesbians we are,*' says Daisy. '*It's a strong strain in everything I've done. I think there were huge – even if unwelcome – benefits for the children in being part of a lesbian family. It gave them an education of what it's like to be on the other side of the fence. Today, where my daughter lives, it's different: there are grandmas, uncles and cousins at parents' day, but in the 1970s to see two flaming feminist women turn up to parents' day with lots of children, it can't have been easy... We never talked about any of this, we just got on, we had four children much the same age so we had to be organised – we had to be a team.*'

The late 1990s, 2000s and 2010s

Men and women's parenting roles have evolved over recent decades and today, many straight couples turn their backs on traditional gender roles. However, in straight couples it is still women who tend to do most of the housework, the childcare and the school drop-offs and pick-ups. It is still women who are more likely to work part-time or take career breaks to care for children than their male partners. So how does this work for same-sex couples? Do they divide along similar lines or do they model a new way of parenting?

Before their son was born, Sara and her partner agreed on their roles, based both on preference and practicality. '*I was the stay-at-home mum,*' she says. '*I was working freelance and my partner was employed on a good salary, so she became the breadwinner, who'd be a parent in the evenings and at weekends.*' So far, so traditional. But roles shifted as their son grew older and as the couple grew apart. '*Now that my partner and I have split up, we have agreed to share parenting 50/50,*' explains Sara. '*She's now changed her work pattern so that she can work two days a week at a local office. We're both clear that we have to put our son's needs first.*'

Victoria and her partner, Nina, also planned a conventional division of roles right from the start. '*We decided that Nina won't work until our son is at school, she runs the house. A friend said to us, "You're the most traditional family I know" – and I'm not sure that was a compliment! I suppose it is ironic that, as a same-sex couple, we have such traditional roles, but I think it's easier to do that when you are both the same sex,*' reflects Victoria. '*You don't have to justify why the man is going to work and the woman staying at home, or vice versa; the person who's most suited to each role can do it, rather than thinking, Hang on, I'm the dad, I should be the one going to work. Straight friends have given us tons of shit about this. The women are very suspicious of Nina's choice to stay at home, as if by choosing what works for us, we are criticising them for being at work.*'

Samantha lives in a part of northern Scotland which is more traditional than many other parts of the UK, and where there are clear ideas of men's and women's roles. '*I'll always remember having a dad, but in my early teens, I noticed little things about him changing – pink slippers under the bed, the hair, the nails,*' she recalls. '*But, I thought, it's the modern world – who doesn't like pink? My dad would take me shopping for clothes. He had a better eye for detail than my mum, he was very "girly" in that way.*'

Her dad was already pushing gender boundaries, but when he started transitioning from male to female, the family were anxious about how their local community would respond. However, despite significant bullying at school, they were accepted more warmly than they expected. Samantha remembers that people still had plenty of questions about living in a family which now had two mums: '*People asked me, "What do you do without your dad? Who will walk you down the aisle when you get married?"*' Not knowing any families with a trans parent apart from her own and having few role models, has given Samantha the opportunity to rethink traditional gender roles and how they apply to *both* her parents. '*When I got married, I came to an arrangement – I asked both parents to walk me down the aisle, it didn't seem fair to single one out. People ask, how will you deal with this or that? You don't know till you come to it, but it works out.*'

Beyond the gender binary

More and more people, including parents, are exploring ideas of gender-fluidity: identifying at different times as male, female, non-gendered and/or any combination of binary and non-binary gender identities.

Naomi identifies as pansexual and her partner, Andy/Mina, identifies as gender-fluid. While they are often perceived as a straight couple, this is not the way they see themselves. With this perception comes an unstated assumption that they will follow traditional gender roles – something they actively resist. '*You're a better parent when you are yourself rather than trying to fit someone else's idea of who you should be*,' explains Naomi. '*We had to decide if we were going to be the conventional couple that people expected us to be or to be ourselves.*'

It's the small things that people notice and comment on. '*In our family, Mummy has short hair and Daddy has long hair*,' continues Naomi. '*When Andy came to the fete at the school where I teach, people asked me, "Why does your husband have long hair?" You could see their brains adjusting to how he looked.*' While sidelong glances, or even open questions, can be annoying, Naomi sees them as an opportunity. '*That's how you change the world, bit by bit*,' she says. '*I had so many fears when I was pregnant. But my colleagues who know are actually envious that I have a partner who has a sense of style, and is interested in shopping and "girly" things. The world is far more tolerant than you think.*'

Naomi and Andy/Mina now face this dilemma with their five-year-old son: how to resist gender expectations while living in a society which reinforces certain gender roles. '*In our family, we are clear that there are no such things as boys' toys or girls' toys, just things we like,*' says Naomi. '*At Pride, our son had a go on the tombola and walked away with a helicopter in one hand and a tiara in the other. He was equally happy with both. He doesn't need "boys' things" or "girls' things", just his things.*'

While they are clear about their parenting approach, they can't help but worry sometimes about how other people see them. The couple have always been open at home about Andy/Mina's fluid gender identity, but are unsure how far to let their son explore his own feminine side, because of what other people might think. '*I find it hard when our son wants to go out wearing a dress,*' says Naomi. '*Especially because I know my parents worry about the example Mina sets. When we're out shopping, how do I tell my son that he's not having the yellow frilly dress that he loves on the rail? But I'm not spending money on something that I'm not comfortable with him wearing out.*'

We might think that other people's opinions don't matter to us, but very often they do. However much we might not want to conform, we don't want our children to suffer for choices we make on their behalf. '*Our son is quite clear who he is and has not realised how uncomfortable that can be for some people,*' continues Naomi. '*For example, he wanted to go to the park in his purple sparkly top and red sparkly "Dorothy" shoes. I said to him, "If you wear girls' clothes to the park, people might think you're a girl – how do you feel about that?" He said, "I don't care." When we got to the park, a boy said, "What are you wearing?" and he said, "These are my Dorothy shoes and they're magic." We understand people might have a problem with that, and we still have some tough years to go. We are trying to give him the language and the understanding to deal with any issues that arise. But I do worry about what people think of me as a parent – will they think I'm pushing a "gay agenda" because I'm not pushing a straight agenda?*'

Working together

Lesbian mum Poppy takes great delight in knowing that her son will see for himself as he grows up that two partners of whatever gender can work as a team. *'Just by being together as a lesbian couple we've fucked up the reasoning that you need a man to do DIY and a woman to cook,'* Poppy says. *'Sometimes she cooks, sometimes I cook, sometimes she cleans, sometimes I clean, sometimes she puts up shelves and changes light bulbs and sometimes I do. We show my son that you don't need a man to put up flat-pack furniture. I can do it all, my girlfriend can do it all, it doesn't matter who does what.'*

Gay couple Dónal and Joseph have always parented as a strong team, especially in the first few difficult months after they brought home their adopted sons. *'Life suddenly became an exhausting blur,'* says Dónal. *'I remember feeling that every muscle was aching from exhaustion. We closed down the hatch and told everyone to stay away to allow the boys to bond with us and settle in.'*

And they did bond, with Dónal at home on full-time adoption leave for six months, and Joseph continuing to work part-time. But when adoption leave finished and Dónal returned to work, their roles suddenly sharply diverged, not because of gender or because of preference, but for practical reasons. *'We swapped roles,'* explains Dónal. *'I returned to work, commuting daily, and Joseph worked part-time and parented. It was horribly tough for both of us. I left before the kids awoke and usually got home to kiss the boys goodnight and read them a story. Poor Joseph was almost a lone parent of two very challenging boys.'*

Nicholas and Michael, as a gay couple whose son was born with help from a surrogate two years ago, had no legal right to time off around the birth. But they were both determined to spend as much of those precious early months with their son as possible. *'We made the moral case with our workplaces that this child needs to be looked after by someone,'* says Nicholas. *'We made a proposal that each of us would extend the non-statutory maternity leave on a pro rata basis, working two or three days a week each.'*

'It was tricky to negotiate,' agrees Michael. *'It took a lot of*

time and stress, it wasn't automatic. But certainly it could have been worse, we got a great package. We asked them to honour the spirit of the benefits package as it would be for a heterosexual parent, despite the law still catching up for homosexuals.'

Unexpected changes in both their jobs meant that this part-time arrangement didn't work out exactly as planned, but Nicholas and Michael remained committed to sharing the time spent bringing up their son as equally as possible – and they managed it. The fact that neither of them gave birth, or had a better claim to parental leave than the other, made this easier to arrange. *'We could split it because we weren't breastfeeding and there were no health implications,'* reflects Nicholas. *'It's helped us both bond with our son and we feel that as a result he has become very comfortable with people.'*

'There's not one of us he favours, it's very balanced,' continues Michael, recognising that the way they developed their parenting roles is quite unusual. *'We were the only gay couple in our NCT group. At the first meeting there were seven women with bumps and blokes next to them, and the two of us. You can imagine the looks we got! These couples, who have become good friends, have approached parenting differently to us. Compared to a division of roles ("Mummy does all this, but Daddy only does this"), it was completely 50/50 for us from day one. We're both male, we both had to juggle things, we had a well-thought-through working pattern – and we were lucky. It wasn't that one of us was back to work after two weeks and the other one had to do everything.'*

Being out and proud as a gay dad

Gay dads can be on the receiving end of sometimes negative attitudes towards men who are hands-on parents, whatever their sexual orientation. *'All the issues I've had have been because I'm a man: a father rather than a gay man,'* insists Felix, who took time off work after his son was born to look after him full-time. He remembers one particularly sticky incident, when he had to get his son's passport photos taken. *'Someone recommended Snappy Snaps, so off we went. We stopped in a café on the way, he was grisly and I tried to feed him. Then he vomited and shat himself. I tried to go and change him, but the* café staff told me I couldn't. I told them I had just seen someone go and change their baby. "Ah, but the changing facilities are only in the women's toilets," they said. We had the whole fight – and still I had to change him in the basement of Snappy Snaps – not an experience I'd want to repeat.'

Some dads find that being the only dad in the toddler group or at the school-gate can be more of an issue than being a gay parent. 'Dealing with the "yummy mummies" at the school gate was tough. It didn't seem to be homophobic, but they were dismissive of our ability to parent. They noticed and commented on all our mistakes,' says Dónal, explaining the pressure he and his partner felt to be 'superdads' to counteract the commonly held belief that men are unable to nurture and do tasks traditionally carried out by mothers. 'I regularly have to firmly remind well-meaning folks that we are capable of looking after our children's needs.'

Richard gave up work when his children were young and became a stay-at-home dad, but he doesn't think that his gender has had any impact on how he is perceived as a parent. 'I don't think as a stay-at-home dad people saw me any differently,' he explains. 'Any negativity just washes off my back anyway, it doesn't penetrate the sphere of my identity. There are more and more stay-at-home dads now, I have straight friends who are, so I don't think it's a big issue now, at least not when others see that your children are happy, well-cared-for, and most of all, visibly loved.'

Finding role models

Gay dads can face questions about whether men can parent as well as women, but lesbian mums can find themselves under scrutiny too, for different reasons. The big question they face, whether during the adoption process, at the fertility clinic or from concerned friends is: what about male role models?

Jenny and her partner, Lucy, used sperm from an anonymous donor to start their family. They would have liked to have used a known donor but it was not possible. They know little about the anonymous donor. Jenny worries about the lack of a male role model for her son and wonders how to fill what she sees as a gap. 'I think after the age of seven, in the stuff I have read, it's really good for boys to have a male role model,' she says. 'There are his uncles, but he doesn't see them regularly enough. We haven't got a plan. I keep hoping we'll meet someone at church, there's lots of gay men there, I keep praying about it. My hope is that he will get into sport and find male mentors there, but it's not quite the same thing.'

Jenny felt that having male role models for her son would become more important as he got older. Paula and Dawn, who parented their foster son for two years on a special scheme for hard-to-place children, felt the same, but for different reasons. Their son came to them, aged nine, after a traumatic early childhood. Paula wonders whether the fact he was placed with a lesbian couple, with no man in the household, has helped him to deal with some of his past experiences and to change his overly sexualised behaviour. 'He struggled more to relate to men. I think he was more competitive with them,' reflects Paula. 'You could see that in how he related to male friends of ours or boys at school. It seemed to us that the men in his previous foster home had found him so challenging that they'd given up. It was still very difficult for him to share Dawn, who was his main carer, with me, but he did let me be a part of his life. I wasn't a threat in the same way as a man would have been.' However, as he approached adolescence, Paula felt he needed a permanent male role model. 'Of course, we would talk to him if he had questions about sex. But by the point of leaving us at 11, he needed a man to show him how to behave in a sexually appropriate way.'

Of all the things lesbian mum Beth worried about when her partner was pregnant, her as-yet-unborn son's lack of male role models ranked high on the list. 'I was obsessed with who would teach him to shave or to use the toilet,' she remembers. 'All the practical stuff about men's bodies. The things we're not quite sure how to do.'

So Beth and her partner, Marie, took steps to ensure they had men around who they knew and trusted to share these difficult questions with. 'We chose two role models for our son who live close and who have or are expecting children. At a pinch, we could ask them...' Marie says, before arriving at the 21st-century answer to every tricky question: '...and if we *really don't know, there's always Google!'*

However, Marie feels that being an LGBT parent means you have to think about gender much more carefully than straight parents do: *'I find the temptation is always there to overemphasise concepts of masculinity in a socially normative way, in order to offset the lack of male role models in our family.'*

Carla and Rita have two adopted sons. As a social worker herself, Carla knew how the adoption process worked and what questions they could expect. *'We did get questions about that old chestnut "how will you make sure your child has male role models?"'* she remembers. *'To be honest, I think that's a perfectly okay question to ask. So we put forward lots of names, including our dads and our best friends.'*

All these experiences go to show that 'male role model' doesn't have to mean 'full-time father'. We are all part of communities in some form, whether it's faith groups or friends, families or football clubs. These communities are where our children grow up, where they get to know adults of all genders and where they work out for themselves who they are and what they want to be.

Shoshana, who was brought up by her two mums, values this multiplicity of role models. *'People often ask me if my parents made sure that my brother and I had men in our lives,'* she reflects. *'We had two strong women raising us, but no fatherly figure to teach us what men should be and do. But if I had a father, there is no guarantee that he would be a good male role model. What if he was overly aggressive, or overly passive? Too loud, or too quiet? How can any single individual provide the sole basis for a child to construct their identity? After all, there is no single correct way of being a man or a woman.*

'Children end up piecing together their own gender identity from the multiple experiences and examples in their life,' she concludes. *'That's why it's good for children to have lots of positive adults around them, and why it's not absolutely necessary for them to have both a female and male parent permanently present. My brother and I may not have had access to a father figure. However, we grew up in a society full of men we could watch, listen to and communicate with, allowing us to assess for ourselves which positive attributes we thought men should*

enact; a glorious pick 'n' mix gender toolbox.'

Bryony, who was brought up by her mum, her mum's female partner and her dad, is often asked questions about the gender roles in her family: *'I'm often asked by curious people "who is the dad?" It's like asking which chopstick is the fork. My mum and her partner have slight differences in their roles and how they parent,'* she goes on to explain. *'But these are more down to their individual personalities than anything to do with their genders or adhering to heteronormative gender roles.*

'This has definitely helped me to question gender roles and stereotypes. The division of labour between my mum and her partner was always equal, and they don't easily fit into most people's gender expectations; they just do their own thing. My dad is straight. He's not a particularly macho man, and he has a deep respect for women. I now live with my partner in a heterosexual relationship and we are both conscious of maintaining equality and balance in our life together.'

Bringing up the next generation

As LGBT parents, most of us have thought long and hard about the implications of having children in an alternative family. We are determined to do what we can to ensure our children grow up happy, healthy and confident in their own identity, even if those around us might regard our family set-ups with concern or suspicion. LGBT people who faced prejudice or disapproval when they were growing up because of their own non-conforming sexuality or gender identity, can be especially determined to bring up their children so that they don't feel pushed into rigid gender roles. But they may also feel protective of their children, and defensive of the families they have created, and at times wish that they could blend in.

So how does growing up in an LGBT family influence children's attitude to becoming parents themselves one day? For, whether we react against our upbringing or seek to recreate the childhood we cherished, we are all influenced by what our parents did, when we decide how to bring up our own children. We asked adult children of LGBT parents whether they think their upbringing has given them a different perspective on parenting, in particular in relation to issues of gender and sexual orientation.

Samantha, whose dad transitioned from male to female when she was in her teens, now has two young children herself. She believes that her experience as a child with a trans parent has influenced her approach to parenting. *'I'm straight and I've been in a relationship for quite a while,'* she says. *'My upbringing has influenced me in how I bring up my children. I've noticed that my son at two is not very interested in "boys' toys" like diggers and mud, he has his Barbies and dollies. He's happy to play with his sister, dressing up or doing my hair.'* Rather than being anxious about this, or trying to encourage her son in a different direction, she takes it in her stride.

This tolerance extends to the way in which she is bringing up her children to treat others. *'My children know not to judge anyone,'* she continues. *'In any family, as long as the children are happy and looked after, they'll be fine. That's my experience and that's what I want to pass on to my children. Just because someone changes their name or their gender identity, it doesn't make them a different person.'*

'Growing up in an LGBT family has influenced how I plan to bring up my future children – how could it not?' says Bryony, who was brought up by lesbian parents and identifies as heterosexual. *'It's not just about attitudes towards LGBT people. My upbringing has also influenced how I would wish any children I have to perceive all minority groups. I want them to have the same open-mindedness about gender and sexual identity that I was entrenched in. I worry that my future children won't have that outlook on life because they will have heterosexual parents, but of course I hope that having homosexual grandparents will still be a big influence on them.'*

Like Bryony, Jacob is in his early twenties and hasn't yet become a parent. He believes that his experience both as the child of a lesbian mother and of growing up as a bisexual man will inform his attitude to parenthood. *'If I choose to have a family of my own I don't think it will be until I am quite a lot older – despite my mum being desperate for grandchildren!'* Jacob says. *'The prospect of having children is quite daunting. Even though I think I would enjoy being a father, I am aware of how stringently gendered childrearing can be and I would have to think about how to raise children without imposing damaging categories of gender on them.'*

Jess is a child of lesbian mothers who identifies as a lesbian herself, and is looking forward to one day starting her own family: *'If you identify as LGBT and are thinking about starting a family but are worried about your child being bullied or being deprived of a biological father or mother... just do it,'* she says firmly. *'Having experienced this upbringing myself, I cannot wait to start on my own LGBT family – which will not only have lesbian parents but also lesbian grandparents!'*

Top tips

1. **Be yourself.** Don't let anyone else impose a pattern of gender roles or expression on you and your family. One of the joys of being an LGBT family is that you can pick and choose from the roles you see around you, and come up with your own as well. With a bit of experimentation, you should be able to find a working pattern, division of roles and parenting style that works for you and your family. You're a better parent when you can be yourself, rather than looking over your shoulder and worrying what other people think.

2. **Surround yourself with role models.** Your children will learn about gender, as they learn about everything else, from many different sources. Much as we might like to think that we, as parents, are solely responsible for shaping and moulding our children, we're not. Books, films, friends, faith and many other influences all play a part in shaping how our children see the world and the kind of people they become. Surrounding them with the greatest range of role models possible will enable them to explore the many different ways to be a man or a woman, or to develop an identity which doesn't conform to a gender binary. It's also helpful to have other families with similar attitudes to gender in your circle of friends, especially if you are choosing a path which challenges social norms.

3. **Stay safe.** It's really important to express yourself and your values, but it's not always safe to do so. There may be times when you have to make a judgement about what's safe and

which battles are worth fighting – both for you and for your children. These decisions are not something to feel guilty about; they are simply part of living as a minority in a majority culture.

4. **Have fun.** From camp to drag, playing with gender roles has always been part of queer culture. It can be challenging, liberating, sexy or simply a chance to let your hair down and have a laugh – so enjoy! Research shows that LGBT parents are no more likely than straight parents to have children than who identify as gay, lesbian, bi or trans. But it does suggest that children in LGBT families may be more open to having relationships with any gender and, if they are LGBT, may come out to their parents earlier.

13

NUCLEAR EXPLOSION

This chapter explores the many different forms that LGBT families can take; and examines what happens when immediate families expand to include donor-dads, co-parents, donors, surrogates, friends, birth families of fostered or adopted children and extended family members.

It's the 21st century. We all know the nuclear family, while still dominant, is in decline. If you take the long view, across time and culture, the nuclear family is the exception rather than the rule. While there are many LGBT families that mirror the traditional nuclear family, albeit some with two parents of the same gender, many do not. Whether this is just tinkering around the edges of the nuclear family, or exploding the whole idea behind it, how can those of us in these new forms of family manage our relationships well and bring up our children to feel secure and loved?

These new models of family, such as co-parenting or families which include a donor or surrogate, are hard to generalise about because each family defines its own roles in its own way. On top of all this, there are new family roles which society doesn't have names for. *'We don't always know how to describe everyone in our family,'* ponders Jessica, whose friend Simon donated sperm to her and her female partner and welcomed them into his extended family. *'For instance, what do you call the mother of the wife of the man who helped you get pregnant?'* she asks.

Jacob has faced similar questions. He has always known his biological father, Paul, but was not brought up by him. *'I really love my relationship with my biological father,'* Jacob says. *'I am also very close to his wife, whom I see as family, but there's no family title for the partner of the guy who donated sperm to your mum, because family as a construct is heteronormative and there often isn't language to communicate that which is outside the norm. But I continue to call her family despite not having an intelligible title to use.'* It isn't the name that matters, it's the relationship.

Friends and other 'not family' relationships

The majority of LGBT people grow up in heterosexual families. While they may be loved and cherished within their families, they have to look elsewhere for a glimpse of their future: to discover what it's like to be part of a minority, to work out how to define their identity and to see how other LGBT people form relationships and families. These are some of the reasons why friendships have traditionally been so important within LGBT communities. Through friendships, we can learn from and encourage each other. We can provide each other with love and support during difficult times. If birth families reject their LGBT children, or fail to welcome same-sex partners or acknowledge grandchildren, new 'families of friends' can stand in their stead.

Some LGBT parents deliberately seek out friendships with other LGBT parents to help their children feel that they belong to a wider community. When she was growing up, Bryony's mum and her mum's partner had a close-knit group of friends who became like an extended family to her. She was always encouraged to look wider than her immediate family for love, support and to enrich her understanding of the world.

'I consider those women and men very much as family. They have all had a massive influence on me,' Bryony says now. *'There's one family where the two daughters were adopted from China, and another where the son was conceived via a sperm donor. Our families are different to one another, but they are all different from the norm, and that is something we have in common. Knowing them has helped me to better understand my own family. The parents in all these families break societal norms in their own, individual ways and are happy being themselves. I suppose there is a culture that we feel we belong to.'*

Friendships between families, or with adults, can be important and enriching for children. They get to see other families close up, and to look to other adults, beyond their parents and grandparents, for a different perspective on the world. The words aren't always there to describe these relationships, but they are still enormously important.

Chantelle and her partner split up when her daughter was just 18 months old. It was a long time before they were able to put the pain of the break-up behind them and resume contact. They could not, and did not want to, create a family relationship after so much time apart, but instead they managed to create something new. *'My daughter's now eight and she does see my ex, but she's not family,'* explains Chantelle. *'She left when my daughter was so young and she went two and a half years without seeing her regularly. That can't be gained back. But they are close now. My ex is like her adult friend, her mate. My daughter stays with her, her partner and their children every other weekend. It's a very busy house and she loves it, it's a different world to our home.'*

Adults who are not parents themselves can also offer the gift of a 'not family' relationship which benefits both parents and children. Ben and Rich are a gay male couple whose lives are full of children, despite – or perhaps because – they are not parents themselves. *'We cherish the time we can offer as godparents, uncles and friends not only to our adult peers, but also to their families,'* says Ben. *'We can provide more time to our goddaughter, godson, five nieces, three nephews and the herd of friends' children, and to the people that change their worlds – their parents.'*

Known donors: Adapting to changing roles

Sometimes friendships end up becoming co-parenting or known donor arrangements. Whether or not friends end up having a child together, the awkwardness and the vulnerability of discussing the possibility can fundamentally change the nature of the friendship.

In their quest to find a known donor, Helen and her partner asked a close, gay friend. It started very promisingly. *'We went to Paris to meet with him and his partner, laughed a lot, drank champagne and agreed we'd have gorgeous babies,'* she remembers. *'Then silence for three months. After which an email arrived saying he was talking to a lawyer as he was worried about "what happens if you want to sue me for paternity payments". I was offended and hurt. Communication broke down. We managed to end it without ending our friendship, but it was a low point because it had seemed so hopeful.'*

There can be a lot of ambiguity around the role of known sperm donors. Are they more donor than dad – or more dad than donor? Many lesbians rely on male friends or acquaintances, straight or gay, to help them start their families, but the role of donors as their children grow up is often undefined, open to misunderstanding and can develop in ways which no one anticipated at the start.

After failing to get pregnant at a clinic using sperm from an anonymous donor, Chantelle asked a close friend if he would help her out by donating sperm. She'd become increasingly uncomfortable with the medicalisation of fertility treatment and hoped to find a way which felt more natural. Her friend said yes, and the insemination worked first time. At the start, expectations seemed to be clear and they all agreed that this baby would be brought up with Chantelle and her female partner as its parents. *'My friend didn't want to be a dad, he wanted to be a donor,'* explains Chantelle. *'He gave me the greatest gift he could have given, but he didn't want to be involved.'*

However, once her daughter was born, the relationship began to shift. *'When he met her he was completely drawn to her, and he became "Daddy",'* continues Chantelle. At the same time their friendship came under increasing pressure. *'My partner and I split up. It was a nasty, difficult separation,'* says Chantelle. *'He became a very important person to me during that time; he was a shoulder, a support. He was very kind and warm. I wanted to give my daughter a sibling, and so I asked him to donate sperm again. That was the trigger for him to run away. It was too much for him and now he has zero involvement.'*

Chantelle is now a single parent with a happy, confident eight-year-old daughter, but dealing with the absence of both her daughter's 'other mother' and the man she knew as 'Daddy' was very difficult for them both at first. *'It was harder for her to have him for a while, and then this absence,'* remembers Chantelle, pondering whether a better-defined arrangement right from the start would have helped them when circumstances changed. *'I've explained to my daughter that he never wanted to be a daddy but a donor, but she remembers a daddy. If I was to do it again, I'd keep it clearer.'*

Like Chantelle, Jackie is a lesbian single mum who asked a male friend, Paul, to help her create a child. *'He didn't want anything to do with bringing the child up,'* she explains. *'I was so desperate to have a child that I said, "I don't want anything, there'll be no commitment and your name doesn't have to go on the birth certificate." So he said okay.'* Once Jackie's son, Jacob, was born, the friendship between Jackie and Paul deepened. As Jacob grew older, Jackie realised that she wanted something more than they had initially agreed: she wanted Paul's name on the birth certificate. But she was worried that asking him would damage his relationship both with her and with Jacob. *'He wasn't that happy about it, but he did it,'* Jackie remembers with relief, and over 20 years later the relationship still holds strong. *'If I made one good decision in my life, it was choosing Paul to be his father. The relationship between them is phenomenal. It's everything I could have hoped for and more.'*

Paul agrees: *'My decision to be a donor has always been rewarding. It was a profound way I could do something positively life-changing for a good lesbian friend, but at the time, it didn't feel as if it would be particularly life-changing for me,'* he says. He now recognises that his involvement has changed over the years, in ways which he did not expect. *'The thanks of a dear friend, and the arrival of a human being were, in themselves, reward aplenty two decades ago. But the myriad of additional rewards over the years has been wonderful too, particularly from being part of Jacob's life and seeing him become the person he is today.'*

The terms 'father' and 'son' don't quite fit Paul and Jacob's relationship. *'I have always been "Paul" to Jacob, although he did (and does) reference me as his dad to some friends,'* says Paul. *'I'm very comfortable with this, and it fits me far better than me self-identifying as his "dad". Being a father is more than the biological act of donation. There is far more of fatherhood that I have not given Jacob than which I have. Our relationship* has grown at a pace that is right for him and me, even if that is slower than some might have chosen. In recent years we have become closer. We text and email regularly. We speak frequently. We share difficulties and excitements and go to occasional gigs.' It's a relationship to cherish no matter what words are chosen to define it.

Lesbian couple Nicki and Rosie had both worked with foster children before deciding to start their own family, and this experience shaped their desire for their children to be able to know their biological father if they wanted. They found a donor by answering an ad in a gay newspaper. However, having no previous friendship to build on meant that each side had to go on trust, a big risk when making such an important decision. Looking back, they can see that there were warning signs from the start. 'We met him once or twice and assumed he was gay, but some of his answers to our questions were a bit oblique,' remembers Rosie. 'We were clear with him that we would be the parents and we didn't want him to be a father. He was fine with that, said he was open either way. Then it went wrong. Once Nicki was pregnant it all changed and he became very intense. He would say things to me like "thank you for looking after Nicki for me". It made us very suspicious, so we stopped all contact. Then we found out he had given us a false address.'

Nicki continues, 'He turned up unannounced on our doorstep two days after I'd given birth and shook my dad's hand, saying, "I'm the baby's father." We told him to stay away. For the next ten years, he just sent cards at Christmas and on our son's birthday. He signed himself by his first name, not dad.'

Despite all of this, their commitment still stood: they would ensure their son could get to know his biological father if he wanted. At the age of ten, their son said he did, so they organised a meeting. This proved to be the turning point in the relationship. 'It's been fantastic since,' says Nicki, still slightly surprised at how well it's worked out in the end. 'He and his wife have become our friends. We see them every four to six weeks. When we go on holiday, they stay nearby. He does things that our son likes to do, like take him fishing. It's been really good for them. Bizarrely it all turned out well.'

Each family in this chapter has had to adapt to change. They may have started out with shared ideas about the role, or not, that a donor would play, but found it didn't work out that way in practice. James is an extreme example: when he agreed to donate sperm to some straight friends who couldn't conceive, he didn't think he'd even be living in the same country as them by the time the baby was born. Instead, they all ended up living in the same house for the next four years.

'*I had planned to stay in the USA for just a year, but I found a long-term job there and decided not to return home to the UK,*' James says now. '*Instead, I continued to live with my friends. They said from the outset that I could be as involved or uninvolved in the child's life as I chose. I accompanied them to antenatal classes and was present in the delivery room when the first baby was born, and again, two and a half years later, for the second. I had no legal rights or responsibilities as a parent and was not named on the birth certificate. But since I was part of the household, it seemed inevitable that I would be involved in our daughter's life once she was born, and to me it felt right too. Initially, we didn't tell anyone other than our families and a few close friends that I was the birth father. I became godfather to the girls, which gave us all a way to describe to others my relationship with them which was truthful, if not the whole truth.*'

The arrangement worked well, but things were set to change again, and again. '*I moved in with the man who became my life partner, though I continued to live close by and to see the girls several times a week,*' continues James. '*Two years after we met, my partner got a job overseas. I did not immediately move with him, because I thought if I left when the children were just four and six, neither of them would remember my ever having been part of the household. So my partner and I had a long-distance relationship for three years before I finally joined him abroad.*' To stay or to go: these were difficult decisions to make, as these different relationships and loyalties pulled James in different directions. Decisions he couldn't imagine having to make when as a 23-year-old, fresh out of university and miles from home, he said yes to a friend's request. But he has no regrets.

'*Back in 1990, I didn't imagine that gay parenting as we know it today would ever be commonplace,*' he recalls now. '*I couldn't conceive of what it would be like to be part of an unconventional family, to live in a home with a baby, or to become emotionally attached to and invested in a child's life.*' And yet this is exactly what happened to him. He continues, '*I also didn't know when – or even if – a long-term relationship might come my way, or how such a relationship might interact with the choices I was making. I learnt that the consequences of such big decisions can be complex, and at times emotionally or practically difficult. Nevertheless, my overarching message would be: despite the uncertainties and unanticipated twists of life, what you have to give – and to gain – by enabling others to become parents, and in some way becoming one yourself, is immeasurable joy. That's been true for me.*'

James has a very close relationship with his biological children, and an ongoing friendship with their parents. By contrast, Victoria's three-year-old son, conceived using donor sperm at a fertility clinic, has never met his biological father. However, this doesn't mean that there is no connection with him at all. Victoria and her partner are open and interested about their son's biological heritage, so they tried to find out more. '*It's not hard to find out who the donor is and who else they have helped to get pregnant,*' says Victoria. '*You have a code number for the donor when you import the sperm. Put it into Google, a few clicks and you're away. We joined a secret Facebook group of people linked to the same donor. You're told there'll be a maximum of ten families using the same donor, but that's just in the UK. So far, we're aware of 58 families worldwide, that may increase, and there will be more we don't know about.*

'*We've told our son that a kind man helped us. He asked if he could meet the donor, we said, "Well, who knows? Maybe one day." He knows his name and has seen a picture.*' While Victoria and her partner do not at the moment want to contact or get to know their donor, they do regard children conceived using the same donor sperm as being related to their son. '*We're now in contact with his half-brothers and half-sisters, his "diblings",*' explains Victoria. '*They are very geographically spread out, so we haven't met any yet. He has seen pictures of them, and we will explain that they are his half-brothers and half-sisters in due course.'*

Surrogates: Building a relationship

A surrogacy relationship is another one that can seem difficult from the outside. But, in many ways, being a surrogate is much clearer than being a sperm donor or donor-dad: most surrogates have their own children already, and will explicitly agree in advance that they won't be 'Mum' to this child. Legal arrangements are put in place before the birth, and finalised after. So to what extent is the surrogate part of the child's family, or the child part of the surrogate's? Many people who've become parents through surrogacy are keen to maintain some connection with the surrogate as their child grows up.

Gay male couple Felix and Evan have a good relationship with Danielle, the woman who carried and gave birth to their son, and hope one day to have another child through surrogacy with her. They also keep in touch with Lou, the egg donor, who is Danielle's cousin's wife. *'It was very important for Danielle as a single mum to involve her wider family, so she was keen for Lou to be our egg donor. It was never something we could have factored into our plans, but for us, it makes the story more complete.'*

The contact they have with Danielle is both for their son's benefit and as a way of thanking her for the gift that she has given them. *'Danielle's a busy woman with four children of her own. She thinks she's done something amazing for us, not that she's given up a child,'* explains Felix. *'When we see her she's not desperate to get her hands on him – she has daughters who'll do that for her! She's interested in him like an aunt would be – I'd say like a grandparent, except our son's grandparents won't ever let him go! It's more intellectual than emotional for her.'*

But how does this work in practice when they live hundreds of miles apart? *'Our ongoing relationship is through WhatsApp, as it was all through the pregnancy,'* says Felix. *'We send pictures, she responds to messages, but we only see her a few times a year. Modern technology makes it work: it's safe, remote, frequent and low-level. We send her a "day in the life" video for her birthday each year, capturing the normal moments of our son's day, none of which would be possible without her. It's a nice annual milestone, even if it's always late!'*

For Nicholas and Michael, another gay couple who become parents through surrogacy, their relationship with Sarah – their surrogate – and her husband and children has become extremely close. It's much more than the occasional message or meet-up, it means a great deal to them all. *'We didn't design it that way, we didn't even know we wanted it,'* says Michael, looking back. *'There's an obvious end goal when you are trying to get pregnant: the relationship you and your partner will both have with your baby. I expected that. What I didn't expect was that the relationship with Sarah and her family would be equally important. They have become part of our extended family. We've not just got a baby now, we've got these wonderful, special people in our life.'*

Nicholas and Michael didn't know Sarah at all before they met through Surrogacy UK. They instinctively got on, spent time getting to know each other and opted for home insemination instead of using a clinic. This, in Michael's words, was *'an awkward process, but possible to get through if you have a good sense of humour'*. This got the relationship off to a good start, but it was a medical emergency in the final weeks of pregnancy that really bound them together. Nicholas picks up the story: *'Sarah's youngest child had been born in ten minutes on the floor at home. There was a real risk to her and the baby if it happened that fast again. So she was admitted to hospital two weeks before her due date.'* But for that first, unexpected week in hospital, Sarah's husband was scheduled to work overseas. Who would look after their children while Sarah was in hospital preparing to give birth to Nicholas and Michael's baby?

'We moved into their house and looked after their kids aged four and six for that week, like being surrogate parents to them,' continues Nicholas, explaining the role reversal which took place that week. *'We did school runs, bath time, everything, it was like a crash course in being a parent. We visited Sarah every day. The hospital made a special arrangement that we could move into a private room on the same floor. So the three of us spent the time there waiting. We became like local celebrities.*

We'd go down to the hospital canteen and random people would come up to us and ask, "Is it a boy or a girl?"

Since then, they've kept in close contact, seeing each other every month. '*We still spend time with her and her children, our son's half-siblings,*' says Michael, illustrating again how Sarah and her family have now become their family too. '*We fell in love with her kids, they know our son and he knows them. We hope that this never changes.*'

Two's company? The joys and challenges of being a multi-parent family

'*I get so many raised eyebrows and puzzled looks when I try to explain how our family works,*' says lesbian mum Yasmin, whose daughter lives with her and her other mother, Lizzie, and spends part of each week with her dads Tom and Damian. '*Once they get it, friends and colleagues seem to think having more than two parents is a great idea, but often I don't bother to explain because I don't have the energy to deal with the questions. I think it must be even more complicated for Tom and Damian. As our daughter doesn't live with them, people can overlook the fact that they are her parents too.*' Yasmin's experience shows that if you choose to co-parent, you need to be prepared: there will be a lot of explaining to do.

The concept of a family with two parents of the same gender is just about possible for most people to grasp. Understanding how a family works which includes three or four parents, from the outset, is another matter. It might look like parenting after an amicable divorce when parents have found new partners: children who live with one set of parents but regularly stay with the other; decisions made jointly between all parents; family get-togethers involving all sides. But there's a fundamental difference between co-parenting where gay men, lesbians or straight people set out to create a family together, and co-parenting after a divorce or separation. It's not an arrangement that is made once a relationship between parents falls apart, it's an arrangement based on friendship, trust and the commitment to build a new kind of relationship from the start.

While UK law is catching up with the reality of same-sex parents, it isn't yet able to comfortably encompass three or more parents who all want to share responsibility for their child's upbringing. *'We wanted all four of us to have shared legal responsibility for our daughter,'* explains Yasmin. *'But Lizzie and I had had our civil partnership before she was born so, in the eyes of the law, only the two of us could be legal parents. Tom and Damian wouldn't be recognised as her parents at all. We agonised about who should go on the birth certificate. We considered saying that our daughter was conceived through sexual intercourse, instead of by home insemination, so that Tom could go on the birth certificate as her biological father, but then Lizzie couldn't have gone on. In the end, none of us felt comfortable with lying to the Registrar about intimate details of our daughter's conception. We did what we could: we changed our wills and made our own written, but non-binding agreement, but it's still frustrating that the law doesn't reflect the reality of our family.'*

It's not only legal structures which don't quite fit. It's squeezing three or four parents into parents' evenings where there are not enough chairs, or squeezing all of your names onto forms where there are not enough boxes. And it's finding the right language and role models to describe your family and the significance of the relationships within it. *'We've got a handful of books about two mums or two dads,'* continues Yasmin. *'But there is little out there to reflect our lives.'* The parent or parents whose children do not live with them most of the time can feel invisible, written out of the neat two-parent family narratives, and vulnerable to not being seen as 'real parents.'

Yasmin and Lizzie wanted to ensure that Damian and Tom were fully involved right from the start. *'They came to antenatal appointments and classes with us. The staff in the delivery suite were fantastic, and they were both in the room with us during the birth,'* explains Yasmin. *'Lizzie and I had paternity and maternity time off work, but Tom didn't feel able to take paternity leave. However, he and Damian were both around as much as they could be, taking some of the strain off us in those first few weeks.'* It wasn't always easy. Amid the constant whirl of feeding and changing, the lack of sleep and the demands of a new baby, each parent also had to make the effort to include and respect the others. *'We experienced conflicting emotions – it felt hard to let go of our new baby, but we really needed the occasional break,'* recalls Yasmin.

'Our friendship has definitely changed since becoming parents,' she continues. 'We are now bound together for life. There's far more riding on this than on a normal friendship. Whatever we do affects them, and the other way round too. It's so hard to talk about this, to be honest we usually avoid it. I think they must find it hard not having our daughter living with them, but they don't say, and we don't want to ask.' The biggest test so far came when Lizzie was offered a job on the other side of the country. 'It would have been a great opportunity for her, for all of us, but we couldn't move away from Tom and Damian. It was painful to say no, but we knew we couldn't take our daughter so far from her dads. It wouldn't be fair. We mentioned it to Damian briefly but we didn't make a big thing of it. What matters most is making this relationship work for our daughter.'

Birth families

When a child is adopted or fostered, their birth family may still be part of their lives. Adoptive or foster parents may have to manage contact between their children and their children's birth families, and to build their own relationship with the birth families. This can be direct contact through regular visits and phone calls, or cards and letters delivered through a third party. It varies from child to child, depending on what the court orders and what's in the child's best interests. These relationships can be tense and awkward, or mutually beneficial. They are another way in which our families, as LGBT parents, break the mould of the traditional nuclear family.

'There's lots of people in our lives who wouldn't be there if we'd had our own children,' reflects Jay, who has a foster daughter and an adopted son. 'We deal with two families who are not our own.' But the relationships which Jay and her partner, Dee, have with the two birth families are very different from each other.

When their son first came to live with them as a baby on a six-month emergency foster placement, Jay and Dee ensured that he had regular contact with his birth family, hoping he would be reunited with them. When this didn't work out, they applied to adopt him. *'His birth family appealed the adoption because we were gay,'* explains Jay. *'That's their right, and you have to respect that, it's their child, but it was hard for us that they could say what they wanted, despite the damage they had caused him.'*

However, the relationship with their foster daughter's birth family is completely different, although this has taken time to develop. *'We are fostering our daughter long-term,'* continues Jay. *'Her mum still has parental consent, and we include her in the decisions we make. We could have applied for permanency, but that would have meant she would have lost her rights, and we couldn't do that to her. We want our daughter to maintain a good relationship with her mum.'*

Jay and Dee nurture that relationship through regular Skype calls, texts and photos, and by ensuring that their daughter meets up with her mum every fortnight. *'Everyone's a winner,'* says Jay. *'Our daughter loves the contact – and she loves coming home. And when she's seeing her mum, it gives us time with our son, just the three of us.'*

Extending families

Creating a non-nuclear family doesn't simply bring one or even two more parental figures into the equation. It can also bring in grandmas and grandpas, aunties and uncles, parents' partners, and more. Just one child can make your family quadruple in size!

It can be lovely – think of all those people to help out! – but it can also be a complex set of relationships to negotiate – think of all those different opinions about how best to bring up the children. Different expectations can easily arise and offence can quickly be caused. It's easy to become defensive of your role and your space, or to unwittingly make someone else feel that their role is being overlooked. These extended family relationships can be most difficult at the beginning, when everyone is settling into their roles, and have not yet got to know each other as family.

Tricia, her partner and their child's donor-dad thought they had it all sewn up. '*When it came to the donor-dad's family, we agreed that contact would be infrequent and through him. It was clear-cut and we loved that our child would have contact with more people who loved him or her... Then my partner became pregnant. Something shifted for me when the realisation hit that my new family wasn't in a queer bubble, but existed in a world where those old labels and family ties had huge connotations.*' Tricia had not realised how excited the donor's parents would be about their new grandchild, and how difficult it would be to work out her own role as a non-bio mum. Talking with their donor provided a way forward, and he agreed to explain to his family more about his, and their, intended roles in the new baby's life. '*While I had the role and no recognised label, he had the label and no recognised role,*' continues Tricia. '*He was worried people would think he was the parent. He wasn't and didn't want to be. He recognised his family's enthusiasm was at times overwhelming.*'

Lesbian mum Jessica has also found that things are rarely clear-cut, as relationships and roles develop over time. She and her partner started their family with help from Jessica's friend Simon, who donated sperm. Soon after their older daughter was born, Simon met his partner, Lisette. '*When they first got together, we asked him, "How does she feel about you having done this for us?"*' says Jessica. '*He replied, "It was one of the first things I told her, because if she's not okay with it, then it's not to be."*' Jessica and her partner went on to have another daughter, again with help from Simon. When Simon and Lisette got married not long after, Jessica, her partner and both girls were in all the family photos.

The extended family has carried on growing. '*Simon and Lisette ummed and aahed for a long time about having children together,*' continues Jessica. '*But now they have a four-year-old and a new baby. The girls think it's fantastic and Simon's ended up with two boys and two girls. There's no confusion – the girls are ours, the boys are theirs, but all together we are a family as well.*' It's not just within the generations, but across them too, that new family ties have been formed. '*For Simon's dad's 70th birthday, we're all going away together: Simon's parents, his siblings and their families and us and the girls because they are his grandchildren, just the same as all the others. The girls are now eight and ten, and our two families go away together all the time, but this is the first time we've been away with the extended family. It has really worked for us, Simon and Lisette are close family friends, and our daughters have three sets of grandparents to love and feel proud of them.'*

Top tips

This chapter's tips deal with building good relationships between co-parents, as well as between parents, surrogates, donors and their extended families.

1. **Be clear at the start.** Talk about the 'what ifs', however difficult it might be to have that conversation. What if the relationship between a couple breaks down, what if extended families want to be more or less involved than you'd like, what if a child asks for more or less contact, and so on. Different things matter to different people: one parent may have strong feelings about names, schools or family life which simply aren't an issue for the others. There are some questions to get the discussion started in the 'Co-parents and known donors' chapter. It's good to get into the habit of talking honestly to each other. Even if you are old friends. Especially if you are old friends.

2. **Check in.** Of course things will change, or be misunderstood, or fail to work out as you hoped. You need to be ready to say when things aren't working, and to recognise the feelings and perspectives of the other parents. This could be as simple as a quick catch-up every few months to stop small grievances or misunderstandings becoming problems.

3. **Keep in contact.** Whether it's WhatsApp or weekends away, keeping in contact is crucial. It can be really hard for non-resident parents to feel included in daily life or decision-making, even when things are going well and even if this is something you have all agreed is what you want.

4. **It's not just about the child.** It's about the relationship between the adults too. Entering into a co-parenting or known donor/surrogate relationship means that the adults

involved now have ties to each other too. If you get on well, this is going to help your child feel loved and secure. If childcare is shared on a regular basis, then decisions about moving house, changing jobs or other major life changes can't be made without discussion.

5. **Be generous.** If you are in a co-parenting, known donor or surrogacy arrangement, it's likely that you, as well your child, will have some kind of a relationship with the other adults' extended families. Family relationships aren't easy, but if you can make it work it can be hugely beneficial all round. This may mean sometimes biting your tongue, blurring the roles a little and being generous.

Special Feature:
Being an ally of LGBT parents

Few straight people give LGBT families a second thought, until a friend or family member comes out or they meet a gay dad or lesbian mum at the toddler group or school gate. Although there can still be hostility, ignorance or prejudice, most people are as friendly as they would be with any other family they meet; the sexual orientation or gender identity of the parents is, or becomes, a non-issue.

However, some straight friends actively choose to become allies of LGBT families, challenging stereotyping and homophobia head-on and educating their children about diversity.

In this special feature, Silvia, who is married to a man and has one daughter in primary school, explains why she believes that understanding and standing up for lesbian, gay, bi and trans rights is just as important for families like hers as it is for those who identify as LGBT themselves.

I wouldn't say we're a LGBT family... I am female and have a male husband, with a five-year-old daughter, who, as far as I can tell, doesn't care one way or another. But I am not interested in labels and I wouldn't call myself straight.

I grew up in a rather backwards, bigoted small Catholic town in Italy and my best friend really struggled to cope with being 'the only gay in the village'. I was the only person he spoke to about the guys he was meeting in secret. I felt bad for him whenever I was going out with someone, because I never had to hide. Having said that, I was the only atheist in the village, and that was considered just as bad, so we were outcasts together.

Fast-forward a number of years, I am living in England with a lovely husband and very precious daughter. I work in the arts and most of my closest friends and colleagues are LGBT. It's unfair to draw comparisons between a small Italian village in the 1980s and London in the 21st century, so I probably didn't need to worry, but I knew I wanted my daughter to grow up in an open-minded environment. I wanted to make sure that should she decide to date a girl one day, it will be just as natural as if she had chosen a boy.

She knows plenty of LGBT couples who we see regularly, and as far as I can tell she sees it as perfectly normal. I read her many children's books which feature LGBT families, although I have struggled with some books where someone in the story has a go at the main characters for being 'different'. Because my daughter didn't see them as 'different', she struggled to understand why someone would be mean to them. I didn't want to put the idea in her head that being LGBT is not 'normal'. She still doesn't know some people have a problem with LGBT people and I'd rather it stayed that way for a little longer, although of course I want her to be aware of the struggle that the LGBT community has faced in the past and still faces today.

I wanted her to know that same-sex couples can have babies too and that some children have two mummies or two daddies. None of my LGBT friends have kids so far, so when she was about three, I started looking for playgroups for LGBT parents. We went to a few sessions which was great. I have taken her to Pride a couple of times and she also came with me to campaign for same-sex marriage outside Parliament, because she wanted our friends John and Jules to be able to get married.

I think it's very important that she is fully aware of how diverse we all are, so that she is never afraid of people who are not like her, whatever she turns out to be like herself. It will be interesting to see what impact this has on her as a person when she is older, but it's reassuring to see that she has been completely unfazed by anything she's come across so far.

Special Feature:
Parenthood is not for everyone

In previous generations, LGBT people have had a huge influence on children and young people without having children of their own. Many have made great teachers, youth workers, aunts, uncles and godparents. Many still do.

However, in recent years something's changed. Now that LGBT families are increasingly visible, assisted reproduction is more widely available and legal protections exist, LGBT people who might never have otherwise considered having children are wondering whether parenthood is for them, facing the social pressure that says parenthood is the only path to fulfilment.

In this special feature, Ben and Rich, a gay male couple in their 30s without children of their own, explain what goes through their minds when someone says, "So, when are you two going to have kids then?"

Ben

'You would make such great parents…' 'You're so good with children, when will you have your own?' 'It's a tragedy for you not to become parents…' These are just some of the well-meaning comments we receive as a gay couple. These are intended to be compliments, and we appreciate the meaning behind them. Yet, if not careful, they can be absorbed with immense pressure and sense of duty.

We love spending time with kids. Both of us have worked in schools, one of us has volunteered with autistic children and the other served as a trustee of a preschool and out-of-school club. We have run Sunday schools, put on arts summer clubs and played five-a-side many weekends with young aspiring future recruits to the Premiership. These opportunities have brought us immense happiness and our lives feel enriched through these experiences. However, believe it or not, parenthood is not for everyone.

Our mantra in life is 'no is not never'. So we are not ruling out the possibility of fostering or even, one day, adopting. However, it's worth considering that it might be the right thing to say no.

Anyone who spends time with children, taking the time to listen to their stories and join in their adventures, will be reminded of humanity's wonderful diversity. We have different needs, different priorities and, perhaps most significantly, different gifts. Anyone who has become a parent will be the first to say how 'life-changing' it is. Therefore it could be as 'life-changing' to decide *not* to become parents.

But why on earth would we reach this conclusion when we have been overwhelmed by generous compliments and love spending time investing in young lives?

As a Christian, I believe the Bible praises the virtues of being part of a family and the role that grandparents, uncles, aunts, cousins, teachers, guides, and, crucially, friends have to play. Jesus greatly valued his birth family, but he also reached out to people who became close friends, including children, of whom he said, 'Let them come to me.' Although not a parent, he realised the importance of investing in, and dare we say learning from, youth.

Do we have days when we question why God would make us 'good with children' but not able to reproduce together? Yes, of course. But what if just one of the reasons God made us this way was to be extended parents to those wonderful children who we are very close to, that we cherish and love unconditionally and can give our time and energy to? That makes a joyful reason for living.

Parenthood can take many forms. Rather than share our personal decision *not* to become parents (remembering 'no is not never', the door's not firmly shut!), it would perhaps be more helpful to say what we *have* become. Knowing we are guests, guides and guardians for our godchildren, or hearing the excitement of our twin nieces saying, 'The uncles are coming!' is priceless. We're delighted with our form of parenthood and in encouraging the phenomenal parenting of our friends and family. We hope that all of us can in some way experience the joy of parenthood – in whatever form it takes.

Rich

My thoughts about parenting have evolved time and again. As a child, remarks by my mother and grandmother that 'he'll make a good father' and 'he'll make a good husband' burdened me with the expectation that I would provide what their own father or husband had failed to be. These thoughts encouraged my adolescent self to remain in denial, and in the closet, for longer. Coming out – much later – was an acknowledgement that I wouldn't have children; that I would not fulfil my parents' dreams.

I came out to myself within a church environment that had nothing positive to say about LGBT+ people and I assumed that children weren't an option. Coming out to others and joining the LGBT+ community, I was introduced at a party to a lesbian couple who spoke frankly of their experiences: 'The first was from a known donor,' they explained. 'Never again! This one's using frozen sperm.' This couple's gift was to move the conversation on from 'could I?' to 'how?'

Ben and I have discussed whether or not we'll have children and, while we won't for now, we love to have a role with the children of friends and family. We've welcomed two godchildren to our extended family and agreed that we would raise them ourselves in the unlikely event of a disaster befalling their mum and dad.

Something new has happened for me in the last couple of years, as more of my LGBT+ peers have had children. Those of us who came out in the new millennium, and dated and committed in the 2000s, are increasingly turning our focus to home and family. Meeting and knowing LGBT+ parents does cause me to think again about parenting.

We LGBT+ people have gained confidence and are increasingly getting on with the ordinary things that others have been able to take for granted. The animal charities are still there at Pride but now we're also reminded that fostering, adoption, IVF, egg and sperm donation and various other means allow us to nurture a child. It is wonderful to see so many LGBT+ people with children at Pride.

Over the years since I've come out, LGBT+ families have moved from the edge of my experience to the centre. I'm excited to play a role in that progress, whether by playing, childminding, talking and listening or even, one day, by parenting myself.

Part Four

Who do we think we are?

14

EVERYTHING CHANGES

Change is part of life: weddings and divorces, births and deaths, new relationships, jobs or locations. These happen in all families. Some are planned, some unexpected, some are for the better and some bring great difficulty and sadness. As well as exploring how to cope with these changes, this chapter also deals with the specific changes that some LGBT families face, such as a parent coming out, transitioning or finding a same-sex partner.

Children are resilient and adaptable but, at times of change, they need more reassurance that they are safe and loved than ever. In the words of Take That, they need to know that 'everything changes but you'.

How to boil a frog

For Susie, it's all about finding the best way to boil the frog. You're probably familiar with the idea even if, we hope, you've never tried it at home: put a frog into boiling water and it will jump out immediately; put in it cold water, gradually turn up the heat and, voilà, you have yourself a boiled frog. It's a grisly metaphor, but it makes sense. Rather than panicking children with sudden, shocking, world-turning-upside-down change, give them time to get used to it gradually. Not by withholding information, but by allowing them space to get used to changes and reassuring them about what will stay the same.

For Susie and her family, it seemed that everything was changing. Her decision to transition from male to female, and her ex-wife's difficulty in accepting that decision, contributed to the breakdown of her marriage. Her children had to get used to their parents no longer living together, as well as adjusting to Dad being a woman. Yet, despite all this change, Susie has always shown her children that the most important things have remained the same. The changes that have happened are a natural continuation of what they've always known.

'It's the boiled frog principle: my clothing got gradually more feminine, I had HRT first, then started living full time as a woman,' she says. 'Throughout, I kept emphasising to the children that I'm the same on the inside. There's always been a family joke that I was gay, and in a way I am, but not that way. I said, "You know I've always been a girly dad, well, now I've been diagnosed..." and I told them, 'I will always be your dad, things won't change that much.' My looks, yes, have changed, but apart from that, not much has.'

Children are likely to take time to adapt to change, no matter how gently and lovingly you introduce it. They may come up with questions and challenges years after you thought everything had settled down. After all, which of us as adults doesn't still blame our parents for something they got wrong when we were kids? But this gradual frog-boiling approach has helped Susie manage the changes and she's been rewarded by hearing her children echo her words back to her. 'They have been very good with it,' she says proudly of her son and daughter. 'They've had their occasional crashes and breakdowns, then they give me a big hug and say, "You'll always be my dad." I blooming love them, they've been great.'

Keep it consistent

Keeping things as consistent as she can is at the heart of Chantelle's approach to parenting, because she knows that her eight-year-old daughter has faced a huge amount of change. 'She had same-sex parents, then a single parent, as my ex left when she was very young. It was the best thing that happened for me because the relationship wasn't healthy. But it was a painful time. It took us about 18 months to adjust after she left. My daughter became fiercely independent very young. She knew two consistent women, then it was just one. There are also carers coming in and out, because I'm in a wheelchair and need carers 24/7. They help me to help her. She attaches to them so when they leave she feels their absence, and this can be a struggle.'

Time has helped. 'It's got much easier as she's got older. Now she solely looks to me for support,' says Chantelle. But it's not just time. Chantelle has taken action to limit change where possible. *'It's imperative that my carers are not nannies,'* she continues. *'They are not there to look after her; they are there to support me to do the physical things. If my daughter fell over, a carer would put her on my knee and get me the cotton wool to mop up the blood. She realises now that I am the consistent person. I try to only hire carers if I know they'll stay. Even if they leave, we maintain a relationship afterwards. After all, I spend more time with my carers than I ever would with a partner. I've also got her a dog, we have a cat who she loves – and I'm not going anywhere.'*

Dealing with divorce and new relationships

Divorce or parental separation can be difficult for children, as well as being painful for the couple involved. But children's experiences can vary enormously, depending on their age, the reasons for the split, how much they are told about what's going on and whether their parents maintain a good relationship after the separation.

JoJo and her partner, Faye, met when they were both single parents, bringing up their children from previous heterosexual marriages. *'Our children were brought into the world at a time when we were married to their dads. They were created out of love,'* says JoJo confidently. *'We both made choices that led to being married with children. We will never regret these choices, as the alternative would be not to have our children. But the longer you live your life trying to ignore who you truly are, the more it becomes an incomplete existence. As time goes on, it becomes something that you cannot ignore and it is not fair to you or the people you love.'*

It was the children who brought them together: *'We found each other at our children's preschool,'* explains JoJo. *'We were drawn to each other and quickly made a connection that neither of us had ever had before.'* But the relationship between JoJo, Faye and their ex-husbands is still strong. Parenting is a team effort. Faye's daughter knows that *'there is a bond and a friendship between her mummy and daddy and that it is centred around her'*; and JoJo has taken care to ensure her four-year-old son and nine-year-old daughter *'know they have a mummy and daddy who love them'.* They are both committed to making sure their children will have the answers they need to any questions about their family. *'We agree that kids need to be told the truth whenever possible,'* concludes JoJo.

Reassuring their children in words and actions that they are loved and cared for, and telling them truthfully about their blossoming relationship, were crucial ways in which JoJo and Faye helped their children to cope with the changes they faced. But they were also aware that their children needed time to adjust: they couldn't thrust too much change on them at once. Not easy to do when you've just fallen in love and want to tell the world! *'At a time when we would have shouted from the roof tops how we felt for each other, we put the needs of our children first,'* says JoJo. *'We had to be as sure as we could be that we were solid and in this together. Our relationship had to be a positive thing, not just for us but for our kids too.*

'We are unashamed to be gay women. However, we need to be mindful of the sheltered part of the country where we are raising our children. We have chosen not to live together at this time, as we feel we can be a family under two roofs. We are both working mums and when life is already this busy we both understand that we need to give our own children our time when we can.'

Meeting new partners

Jasmina's only daughter was three when her husband left her. Jasmina came out when her daughter was 12 years old, but it was still just the two of them. That all changed when Jasmina met her new partner. *'When my daughter was 15 I entered my first lesbian relationship,'* says Jasmina. *'She found this difficult, as did my partner, who was not used to children. Then, two years later, my partner came out as trans and we had another part of the journey to get used to.*

'The first challenge was that my daughter was jealous of my partner. My daughter was used to having a monopoly on my attention and felt she was losing mum. My partner didn't really get this. I felt torn between the two of them. This was one of those things which was not to do with sexuality, but something which most single parents go through when they start dating again,

particularly if their partner doesn't have experience of children. This took time for me to realise, because I initially thought the "no public affection" rule my daughter imposed on us was to do with our sexual orientation.'

It was time, and gritted teeth, that allowed the relationships to grow smoother. It got easier once Jasmina told both her daughter and her partner that, while they were each important to her, they both had to give and take. '*It also helped,'* remembers Jasmina, '*when one of my daughter's friends made it clear that she felt it was okay for me to be happy and that my daughter should give me a break.'*

Her daughter has now graduated and moved away, giving Jasmina some distance to ponder on what, if anything, she could have done differently. '*As I reflect on the journey we have been on as a family, I'm aware that we have all done and said things we probably wish we hadn't, as well as things we are glad we did,'* she says. '*That's the same in any family. Now, my partner and I are happy and my daughter feels part of our family – even if she wishes we were a little more normal sometimes. I'm quite happy to settle for that.'*

When Jay and Dee got together, Dee also already had two children from a previous marriage. Jay knew it would take time for the children to trust her. Her acceptance into the family would be on their terms, not hers. '*When I moved in with Dee and the children, they were already a family unit. I had to appreciate that, I couldn't expect them to fit in with me,'* she says. '*I knew her children came first, and the children knew that too. It was difficult for them to go from a traditional family, with no issues about friends coming round, to an untraditional family where maybe they felt they couldn't be so open at school.'*

Fourteen years later, the relationships are rooted and flourishing. Jay has consistently been there for the children during their childhoods, cheering them on at sports days and picking them up from school. Now they are older, she's on hand to answer questions about periods and how to chat up girls. '*They don't call me mum. I'm not their mum, but I am still important in their lives,'* she explains with pride. '*They get me Mother's Day gifts, I don't ask them to, but they do. We've brought them up to be very open and not to label people. Our son has gay friends and goes to gay clubs, it's great. Not all kids – or adults – have that openness. He says he wants to find a relationship like ours one day – when you hear that, you know you've done it right!'*

It can take your children time to adjust to a new partner, as Jay and Dee's experience shows. It can also be hard for a new partner to adjust to family life. After a difficult break-up with their dad, Mel was worried about the right time for her new girlfriend to meet her daughters. '*I was with her for about three months before I started introducing her to the girls*,' she says, but the reality of Mel's family life was too much for her girlfriend to cope with and she pulled away, something which Mel looks back on with regret. '*She was brilliant with them, but it was too much for her. It's tough for them now as they miss her too. I put them through all of that for nothing.*' Since then, Mel's tried to overcome her own hurt, so that her daughters can learn that the end of a relationship does not have to be the end of the world. '*Since we split up, my ex has been round a couple of times for dinner. It's important that the girls can see that we are still friends. I didn't want them to see anything negative or unpleasant.*'

Rituals and rites of passage

Sometimes those new relationships can blossom. So much so, that gilt-edged invites are sent out, outfits are bought, vows are written and wedding bells rung. While seeing a parent get married or enter into a civil partnership is another change, this public rite of passage can help children to accept a new partner, recognise the happiness that they have brought to the family and express their own love for them. This was the case for both Jasmina and Lynn.

Jasmina's daughter's relationship with her new partner got off to a rocky start, but when Jasmina and her partner held a thanksgiving service to celebrate their civil partnership, it was important to them both for Jasmina's daughter to be their bridesmaid. Yet they were wary of approaching the subject, worried that she would say no. '*She was 19. We were clear this had to be her choice*,' says Jasmina. '*If she didn't want to do it, we had to accept that.*' But their fears were not realised. She said yes on one condition: that she got a new dress for the day.

That was easily done, and now Jasmina can look back on a great day, shared with the two people most important to her.

Like Jasmina, Lynn was in a heterosexual marriage with children before she came out. After surviving a difficult divorce, she never expected to live with another person or to get married again. *'I had no idea I'd meet someone and fall in love, for the first time really, so fast,'* she says. *'Or that it would be someone who lived on the other side of the world.'* Lynn's whole vision of her future changed rapidly when she met Glenys, an Australian on holiday in the UK. Thankfully, Lynn's three grown-up children, a son and two daughters, clicked with her new partner straight away. *'Glenys met my older daughter, who thought she was wonderful from the word go,'* says Lynn. *'In fact, it was a bit annoying: she liked her so much that she sat with us for the whole of the first evening that Glenys came round, when I'd planned for it to be just us two!'*

A turbulent few months followed: the couple tried to manage a long-distance relationship while both working full-time on opposite sides of the globe, with limited funds for plane tickets. Then Lynn was diagnosed with breast cancer. Glenys and the children rallied round to support her, using Skype to share news between Scotland and Ireland where two of Lynn's children now lived, her hospital bed in England and Australia where Glenys was still living.

The eventual good news of Lynn's recovery was soon followed by more good news. *'Last year, we got married at the British Consulate in Australia,'* smiles Lynn. *'I asked both girls if they'd like to say a few words at the reception. My younger daughter said yes, but my older daughter's quite shy, so she said she wouldn't. The reception came and after the planned speeches, Glenys asked if anyone else wanted to say anything. My older daughter came up to speak. I was so thrilled, you could see how frightened she was, how terrified by speaking in front of so many people. She said it was not like welcoming Glenys into the family, because she was already part of it. I knew that my older daughter really didn't like speaking in public, yet she did it in front of all those people that she didn't know. That meant such a lot to me.'*

By contrast, Nicki and Rosie had been together for 22 years

before they celebrated their civil partnership. During those 22 years, they'd planned having children together, brought up their son and daughter together, faced challenges together and built a strong family together. The civil partnership wasn't going to change anything. Except, somehow, it did.

They had recently been going through a hard time. Rosie had been diagnosed with breast cancer and their son was struggling at school and at home, taking it out on his mothers with insults and homophobic language. Nicki explains what she thinks was going on, '*His whole world was turning upside down. We had to talk with him about sticking together as a family, otherwise we'd be destroyed. We're not religious, but we do think it's very important to create our own rituals. The civil partnership, when our son was 12, made a lot of difference to him.*' Perhaps there was something about seeing so many people recognise and celebrate the strength and commitment of his parents' relationship that helped him feel more secure. He had tested the boundaries and they had held firm. And it was quite an event by all accounts. '*We started off thinking we'd have two witnesses and a couple of friends,*' admits Nicki. '*We ended up with 150 people – family, friends and work colleagues!*'

Regular rituals can be just as important as one-off rites of passage in cementing family relationships during times of change. Jay and Dee's household includes Dee's two birth children, their adopted son and foster daughter, as well as two dogs, a cat and a parrot. Over the years, it's also included other foster children or children staying on respite breaks. There's always lots going on, and plenty of change to cope with, but Jay has found that something as simple as a regular family meal can keep everyone connected: '*We always have dinner all together once a week, at our older son's flat or ours or we go out. We catch up and have a natter, each week without fail. Every night we eat at the dining table, it's a time for everyone to catch up. Even our foster daughter, whose communication skills are very limited, has a go and joins in, listening and laughing.*'

When LGBT families break down

Janice and her partner were the first same-sex couple in their local authority to adopt. They were well-supported by friends, extended family and social workers when they adopted their older daughter. They went on to have a civil partnership and adopt a second daughter. It all seemed to be going so well. '*Sadly, while on adoption leave, my partner spent a lot of time with another gay mum,*' says Janice, explaining how their relationship began to unravel. '*After nearly ten years together, she left me. To say I was devastated would be an understatement.*'

Then began the tough job of working out how to parent together once the relationship had fallen apart. '*I was kind of in a "dad" role, as the one who hadn't taken adoption leave and was working full time,*' continues Janice. '*But there was no way I was going to miss out on my girls. I insisted we split our time with them 50-50. I was scared about how I would cope – but I did.*'

Three years on from their split, Janice believes the children have adjusted well because she put her devastation aside and got on with doing what was best for them. She's matter-of-fact about the situation she found herself in, and has no time for blame or regret. '*Separation and divorce can happen to anyone, LGBT or heterosexual,*' she advises. '*Like all families you have to take what life throws at you and make the best of it. My ex and I now co-parent as best we can. We even spend Christmas Day and birthdays together.*'

From the children's perspective, separation or divorce can raise difficult issues when you have a biological connection with only one of your parents. Shoshana was brought up by her two mums. She recognises from her experience that the significance of non-biological relationships is often overlooked.

'*When I was fourteen, my family's collective household was disbanded,*' she says. '*We moved out of our single end-of-terrace house, into two separate smaller ones. My brother and I moved between the two houses, dividing our time equally between our two mothers. We adapted quickly. Apart from the occasional realisation on a Sunday evening that all of my school shirts were at the wrong house, I was quite content.*'

However, Shoshana was faced with assumptions that surprised her. '*On finding out that the family had separated, teachers and family friends would ask if I was living with my birth mother, or even whether I still saw my non-birth mother,*' she explains. 'The assumption they made was that the kids belonged with the woman who had carried them in her womb for nine months. Much less thought was given to the years of carrying us as babies, toddlers and young children which followed, which were split equally between both of our mums. The physical separation of our household meant that people who'd previously grudgingly accepted our family, could now openly question our relationships. As though 14 years' worth of love vanished in one day, one moving van, one mile's distance.

'My mums might not have been living together as a couple any more, but they continued to co-parent us. They made sure they were always on the same page, and that we weren't able to play them off against each other. But more importantly, even if they hadn't remained cordial, even if they'd disputed custody, even if I'd moved halfway across the world and not seen my non-biological mum for years, she would always be 100% fully, completely my mum.'

Adoption and fostering

The principles in this chapter of consistency and reassuring children of how much they are loved are all part of how adoptive and foster parents have to approach bringing up their children. Most adopted or fostered children will have experienced huge amounts of change in their short lives. Carla, a social worker and mum of two puts it starkly: 'For our boys their whole life changed in one day – all they knew, where they lived, who they lived with, it all changed. Only being with each other was the same.'

As an adoptive parent or foster carer, you need to help your children to understand and cope with those changes, while coping with enormous changes in your own life too. It's hard to do that alone, which is where the support of partners, friends and family comes in.

'The whole process is so intense,' says Alison who adopted a 16-month-old with her partner last year. 'It's strange to say, but the first two weeks he was with us was the worst point. Oh my God, it was so hard. We thought, What have we done? Should we have got another dog instead? And then we felt so guilty about feeling that. While I was on adoption leave, my partner *was promoted. So she's had to cope with a new job, a new child and a new crying, moaning partner – she's had to do far more adaptation than me!'*

Bronwen, whose daughter was nine at the time of adoption, felt much the same way. *'The fear of not bonding and of worrying about not loving my daughter took months to resolve,' she recalls. 'Now I can recognise that I suffered from post-adoption depression in that first year – I lost two stone in weight (the anxiety weight-loss plan!), ticking all the boxes in the handy list published in* Adoption Today *magazine. I had been unaware of such a condition. Not knowing that the feelings I had were normal added to my sense of anxiety. I felt I couldn't discuss them with social workers in case they said the placement wasn't working.'*

As a single parent, she had no partner to cry and moan at, but her mum provided a helpful sounding board and source of advice for coping with the changes. *'My mum pointed out that there was no going back. I wouldn't have a say if this was my birth child, so decision made – get on with it! This was actually very helpful as I accepted the situation. My daughter and I are now very securely attached – I cannot imagine my life without her.'*

The experience of adopting or fostering a child, and the huge changes and challenges that brings, can put pressure on relationships between partners and within families. This is certainly what Dawn and Paula found when they fostered a hard-to-place child on a two-year placement. *'At first we thought, if we fall in love with him, they'll just say he can stay,'* says Dawn. *'But we came to see why there was a time limit, as we couldn't sustain it any longer. We did our bit with integrity and heart, but the impact on our relationship was enormous. I can't break it down, whether it was parenting or parenting that particular child: his personality and his needs meant he was enormously difficult to live with. There was so much tension, we've never argued so much. We heard that from so many foster parents, even ones who said they'd never argued before.'* Paula adds, *'After he left us, we needed time to rest and to reassemble our relationship.'*

For Carla, both family support and friendships have been

important. Although some friendships, when people failed to grasp that adopted children have specific needs, have been lost, others have been gained. '*As adoptive parents, we have to parent our children differently,*' she explains. '*This has caused difficulties with some friends. Some friends have found our way quite challenging and have buggered off. Friends with birth children don't always understand, they say, "Why don't you use the naughty step or timeout like we do?" but we can't, because our children experience it as rejection. That has been the biggest cause of contention. So, while we have old friends, it's been really important to make new ones, friends who have children, and friends for our children.*'

Telling the story

Whether you face a break-up or bereavement, whether your relationships are amicable or strained, whether change is constant or occasional, whatever kind of change you face, how you frame it and explain it makes a difference to how easy it is to accept.

Susie and her ex-wife had totally different ways of framing her transition and the impact on the family: '*My ex told people that I was having a nervous breakdown, not that I was sorting my life out.*' Instead, Susie framed the changes as positive, as much as she could. This meant that Susie was open to seeing good results, even ones that she didn't expect. '*Most people think about the physical changes of transitioning, but these are nothing compared to what goes on in the mind. I've found more inner calm. Before, it was like having a mains buzz in my head all the time and now someone's switched it off,*' she explains. '*It's transferred to my parenting. My children have said, "We prefer you like this, you're not angry, stressed, shouty Dad any more. If there's a problem, you talk about it." I discuss things more now, I'm calmer than I was and the kids know that.*'

Bryony and her family have also developed language and metaphors to positively frame their family situation. Bryony was brought up by three parents since she was five: her mum, her mum's female partner and her dad. The image that Bryony's found most helpful to explain her family is that of tessellating shapes, which fit together to form patterns that can change and re-form while the shapes themselves remain the same. *'We often describe ourselves as a "tessellating shape", because we fit together, and we are also adaptable,' she says. 'We adapt with the times and changes – such as when I went from staying at my dad's house every other weekend as a child, to spending an evening a week with him (but going home again), to meeting up with him whenever we felt like it when I was a teenager, to now when I see him as and when, just as I see my mum and her partner. We have adapted to include past partners of my dad's and to having family members and friends come to stay with us for periods of time for various reasons. Our relationships change, but we always tessellate.'*

Top tips

1. **Take it slowly.** If you are a parent who first comes out once your children are older, you will have to come out to them too. You might have been thinking about coming out for a long time and be quite used to the idea, but it may never have crossed your children's minds before that their mum or dad could be LGBT, especially if they don't already know many LGBT people. You may have to hold back some of your initial enthusiasm, excitement and desire to be out and proud, until they have had time to adjust.

2. **Be honest – but positive.** Every change has positive and negative aspects. However, even positive changes for parents, like transitioning, coming out, adopting children or forming a new relationship, can be unsettling for children at first. And, let's be honest, it can be an emotional roller coaster for parents too. You might think you've explained everything clearly to your children, but unspoken fears or misunderstandings can remain. As parents, we need to walk alongside our children through the changes, recognising that they may struggle, and be prepared to answer their questions honestly.

3. **Remember you are not the only one.** Regardless of whether it's an opposite-sex relationship or a same-sex one, or whether your children are toddlers, teenagers or adults themselves, introducing your children to a new partner or setting up a new home with them can be challenging.

Even if they get on well, there will be a time of transition, as children work out how to share their parent with someone else and as the new partner finds their role in the family. Realising that this is not just an issue for LGBT parents, but for all kinds of parents in this situation, can make it easier to manage.

4. **Get the support you need.** Times of change can be tough. Even more so when you have to help your children come to terms with it, as well as dealing with the impact on you. While many LGBT parents have supportive families and friends who will rally round in a crisis, others find that if a relationship breaks down, if they move to a new area, or if their family or friends are not accepting of LGBT people, they feel isolated and cut off from former sources of support. Even if it's just one friend you can call, one family member who supports your decisions or an LGBT support group or helpline, make sure you have someone to talk to. Many contributors to *Pride and Joy* remember individuals who have helped them get through tough times many years before with affection and gratitude.

15

STAYING GAY

It's common for parents to feel that their own identity has disappeared once they have children. But it can be even more difficult to maintain an LGBT identity as a parent. This chapter explores how to 'stay gay' in a world of nappies, toddler groups and family-friendly pubs.

All of us hold a multiplicity of identities, and at different moments of our lives, different identities will come to the fore. For many LGBT parents, there will be times when their LGBT identity is the most important, and times when other identities will come first.

For trans people there is a choice, between whether to share information about their trans history, or whether to live in their true gender and not reveal to others that they were assigned a different gender at birth. Mum of two Susie explains her decision, '*You see a lot of "career trans" people, who go on about it. I did it to feel better and to get on with my life, not to be a feature. No one at work knows*.' In her daily life, it is Susie's lesbian identity rather than her trans history that matters to her: '*I go to a lesbian social group and find it helpful to chat with the other women there about our children, but I am not out there as trans*.' Katie and Jim have always been open about Jim's trans history with their children, but not outside the family: '*When we started going out, Jim had been living as a man for 20 years*,' says Katie. '*Although Jim is not public about being trans, we decided to tell our children from an early age*.'

For other parents, even if they are out as LGBT, their identity as a parent becomes more important than their sexual orientation or gender identity. '*How will we survive early parenthood?*' was the big question for bi mum Marie, remembering the huge life changes that came simply from becoming a parent. '*For the first few years, the gay identity thing was much less important than the identity of being new parents.*'

LGBT people who start their families after coming out may struggle to keep up with the friends they had before they had children. Not only has your pace of life changed, but your priorities have too. '*Over one night, we went from being gay men about town to being fathers of two very active, traumatised, scared boys. We were fathers, Daddy and Papa, but without a sexuality any more,*' says Dónal, gay father of two adopted sons. '*Most of our gay male friends slowly vanished. None were ever dismissive or anti-child, it was just that we were no longer available to hit the town on a Friday night, and had to meet for lunch rather than dinner. Without realising it was changing, we suddenly discovered that our closest friends were now other parents, mostly heterosexuals.*'

If you have spent years planning how to have children as an LGBT person, it is not surprising that once you become a parent, this becomes a hugely significant part of your identity, at least in the early years. Being an adoptive parent or foster carer, with its particular experiences and challenges, can be as significant, or more so, than being LGBT. '*We have been invited to be part of a number of LGBT parenting groups but tend to avoid them,*' says Dónal, thoughtfully. '*The issues faced by biological parents are quite different from the issues faced by foster carers or adoptive parents. I find I have far more in common with heterosexual adoptive parents, of either sex, than biological lesbian mothers.*' However, Dónal and his partner did join a regular gathering of LGBT adoptive and foster parents and, looking back, he can see the difference this group made to the whole family: '*We got to spend time with other queers who had made a similar journey and who were dealing with issues like insecure attachments, trauma and loss. I can't put a value on this amazing support. The boys loved it and it was helpful for them to meet other kids from families like ours.*'

Bronwen agrees. Last summer, she and her 11-year-old daughter packed their tent, sleeping bags and wellies and headed off to New Family Social's annual camping weekend. '*Attending the weekend was incredibly liberating and positive,*' says Bronwen. '*To meet so many LGBT parents and foster carers was brilliant. For my daughter to realise she was not the only older adopted child (until then, we'd come across an awful lot of babies but not so many teens) was very affirming for her too.*'

LGBT parents' groups: The good, the bad and the ugly

Becoming a parent was a huge change for Jessica and her partner, but they went through this experience alongside many of their closest friends. It was a time when their friendships with other lesbians deepened, rather than drifted apart. Jessica explains, '*We've been part of a lesbian social group for a long time. Lots of our friends there now have children. Those long-term friendships are so important to us. There is so much support around us that often we don't even notice. There are lots of lesbian parents near us, even in our village. I can't imagine feeling unusual.*'

Jessica and her partner value the friendships they have with other lesbian parents, but other parents are more interested in the benefits LGBT parenting groups bring to their children. Jenny and her partner take their son and daughter along to one such group, not to get support for themselves, but because they want their children to see that there are other families with two mums. '*Just because people are lesbian and have children doesn't mean you've got anything in common with them,*' says Jenny. '*What matters more for us, because we're older parents, is not having* our *parents around to help. In the early years, we could have done with much more practical support, never mind the LGBT stuff. Who cares about that? In this day and age I just don't think it's all that significant. It's about being a parent – frankly, what we needed most was someone to come over and babysit!*'

Groups vary, and unfortunately not everyone has positive experiences of them. Single parent Tony did not. '*Sexuality for me has always been a sliding scale – or a slippery slope depending on how you look at it,*' says Tony, who separated from his wife 12 years ago, shortly after their son was born. '*I can't define it, and I'd be happier if others didn't feel the need to – save the labels for presents and for small minds that need to put everything in a box.*' But now '*boxed and labelled as a gay dad*', Tony was left with numerous questions about how to manage his relationship with his son. He went in search for answers and ideas, starting with a gay dads' support group: '*This was an interesting experience – a group of dads who were gay that slept with men behind their wives' backs for the sake of keeping the family together. I'm not being judgemental but... this just wasn't what I was looking for. So I searched for other groups, for books, for any resources – and time and time again all I found were resources for mums.'*

So why seek out an LGBT parents' group? The answer is twofold. Firstly, to maintain your identity and find mutual support for the specific joys and challenges you face as an LGBT parent. Secondly, to provide an environment for your children where their family is seen as 'normal', so that when they say 'but no one else has two mums', you can simply point out all the people they know who do. '*I joined a group of LGBT parents because I wanted my daughter to know she's not different – and I wanted that for me as well*,' explains lesbian mum Chantelle. But she found, like with any group, it took time to build genuine relationships with others. '*I started going along with my partner. After she left me, I went into a very dark place. It seemed like the other parents were all couples. I just wanted to hide. But when another parent said very openly that she'd split up with her partner, I realised there were a lot of single gay parents in the group. I was feeling abandoned, so I made an assumption that everybody else was happy. But in the group there were all aspects of parenthood – now I realise that everybody is completely different and that's what makes it so wonderful. I want my daughter to meet all kinds of people and to be free to choose how she is herself.*'

There's something very powerful about meeting others with whom you share a common identity or experience. There are things you don't have to explain or justify. You can be yourself. Yet some groups can be experienced or perceived as *lesbian* parenting groups, rather than groups that include gay men, and bi and trans people whose lives 'look straight'. '*I'm coming out of a stage where my primary identity was "mother" and I didn't really have an outlet for any of the other aspects of my identity*,' says bi mum of two Rebecca. '*My sexual orientation is just one small aspect of who I am, but it's an important one* nonetheless. I'm acutely aware of my "passing" privilege, and I know that if I were in a same-sex relationship, I'd face different (and tougher) challenges. So that's why I've not really sought out LGBT parenting groups – I'd feel that we weren't facing the same challenges and I would be worried that I wouldn't be welcome.' Naomi agrees: 'I can't really go to lesbian parenting groups, because I've had my baby with someone who's biologically male,' she says, 'but I don't fit in with straight groups either. I'm still trying to work out how my identity fits into things.'

However, Rebecca has been lucky enough to stumble into friendships with other LGBT parents. 'During maternity leave I came out to another mum who I'd made friends with,' she says. 'I was over the moon when it turned out she was also bi. It felt like coming home – someone who could relate to me as a whole person.'

Developing an LGBT identity

Parents who come out later in life, once their children are older, face different challenges. For them, it's not about maintaining or reviving a connection to the LGBT community, but establishing that connection in the first place. Exploring the scene, making friends, finding a partner – all this is new, exciting and often nerve-wracking. But the same old routines of childcare and the school run carry on regardless. It's not like coming out when you are young, single and (reasonably) carefree.

The practicalities of separating from her husband and helping her daughters cope with the change meant it took Mel some time before she could start exploring her new identity and looking for a partner. But, sadly, her experiences of being out as a parent in the LGBT community have not always been positive: 'I joined a dating site, but I had to block some people because I was receiving abusive messages, like "what gives you the right to look for a relationship when you have children?" I'm very honest in my profile that I'm a lone parent, I have two girls, one with special needs. It's only fair to be upfront about it. One or two people do keep in touch and send me messages from time to time, which gives me the adult conversation I need.' She has also struggled to meet other LGBT parents. 'The hardest thing is not having other similar families to meet up with and relate to,' she continues. '*I still don't know any other lesbian and gay families. I think there used to be a group nearby, but it closed down due to lack of interest.*'

Lynn's children were in their teens by the time she came out, and old enough to offer her support as she tentatively found her way in the LGBT community. Lynn's older daughter's coming out as bi was an important moment in Lynn's own coming out process. '*When she came out, and I saw she was happy, I think I was jealous,*' says Lynn. '*I wonder if that was the start of the process for me. Before I came out I didn't know any other gay families, so part of coming out was simply meeting other lesbians. I went along to a lesbian group, but arrived far too early because I was so nervous. I texted my daughter, telling her how nervous I was. She texted back to say it would all be fine – and it was. It was so friendly, you could chat to anyone and someone always kept an eye out for new people.*'

Pride and prejudice

Some parents, like Sally, find their enthusiasm for Pride has grown since they have had children. '*I'd been on Pride marches before, and felt the heady glow of walking with people "like me", full of courage, bravado and, yes, pride,*' she says. '*But this year I experienced it anew: I walked with my daughter. Granted, she slept for most of it, but walking through the streets of my city with friends and thousands of others, with an estimated 75,000 looking on, felt different this time. I was not only proud to be gay, I was proud to be the mother of my beautiful little girl. To be both of those things publicly still feels a little radical. At Pride, it felt wonderful.*'

At Pride, it can be a thrill to see your family reflected in the other same-sex couples marching with buggies or clutching toddlers with ear defenders and rainbow face paints. But it can be hard work, especially with little ones. The crowds, the heat (or the rain), the need for loo breaks and snack stops, the waiting around, the noise, the drunk people, the sheer amount to carry. Any trip out of the house with very young children can be hard, but a trip to Pride can feel overwhelming.

This hassle, and the lack of family-friendly facilities, has put some LGBT parents off the bigger city-centre Prides, despite being regular attenders before. Chantelle and her daughter go to a Pride at least once each year but, despite living close to the capital, they don't go to Pride there any more. '*I used to love it when London Pride was in the park, you could just wander around seeing a bit of everything,*' explains Chantelle. '*In the streets it's harder. When I took my daughter to London she was very young and I wore her in a sling. People got close to her with their cigarettes and I just didn't feel Pride had the space and was the family-orientated experience it used to be.*' But Pride remains an important part of Chantelle's identity: '*It's the chance to celebrate who you are and the joy of being who you want to be.*'

Pride doesn't have to be the all-out, thousands-strong, rainbow-coloured extravaganza that it is in the big cities. For parents like 20-year-old Poppy, who live outside the main gay centres of London, Brighton and Manchester, local Prides provide a place of acceptance and friendship, and rare visibility for LGBT relationships in their neighbourhoods. '*I volunteer for Pride in my town every year,*' she says. '*There's a handful of lesbian volunteers; they're all older than me. I get so much support from being with them, and from straight allies too,*' she explains. '*I can walk along holding hands with my partner and my son, and no one bats an eyelid. People smile at us as we walk through town, just like we're normal people, because we are.*'

Rebecca's bi, happily married to a man and has two young daughters, but feels that '*becoming a parent compounded my lack of visibility as LGBT. People tend to assume I'm straight anyway, and the addition of children just adds another layer of assumptions.*' So being visible at Pride is especially important for her, even if her children are less impressed: '*I go every year. It's the one time in the year I'm unambiguously and publicly identifying/identified as queer. I've taken my eldest daughter along as a baby, but she's not that interested in attending now she's older, despite my attempts to bribe her with a rainbow fairy outfit.*'

Dónal's return to Pride after a 13-year absence, and his discovery of a new group of queer friends and allies came almost by accident. When the Irish government announced that the electorate would have the opportunity to change the

Constitution to make marriage genderless, in other words to allow for 'gay marriage', he knew he had to get involved in the campaign. He threw himself into the struggle for justice alongside members of LGBT communities, family members of LGBT people and lots of straight allies. The family joined the umbrella organisation Yes Equality and started to canvass in their local area.

'From the start our kids were involved, and we found a new group of queers of all sexes and gender identities to call friends,' enthuses Dónal. 'It's been wonderful, and to cap it all, the people approved the amendment by a landslide! I was involved in reviving the LGBT Pride march in Dublin in the early 1990s, and look forward to taking part again after such a long time. Now that the Marriage Equality amendment has been carried, the atmosphere will be amazing. This time we're taking the boys too.'

What about the children of LGBT parents? We might love Pride (or hate it) but how do our children experience Pride? When they are small – and they have no choice if we take them – we can help them find the fun. Dodgems, face-painting, tombolas, free sweets and stickers are all Pride highlights for children whose families contributed to this book.

Both Miriam and her ex-husband identify as LGBT and their nine-year-old daughter is a big fan of Pride. 'We've been for the last few years,' says Miriam. 'Her dad's company has a float, so I go to watch with her, pass her to her dad to join the march, then pick her up at the end. She adores it all.'

Later, when children are a bit older, with their own social lives and group of friends, they'll probably be less interested in coming to Pride, or hanging out with their parents at all. But by the time they're adults themselves, like Bryony or Shoshana, many will be back, with fond memories of their early Prides.

'We went to Pride as a family a couple of times with a community of family friends. I have also been as an adult with my boyfriend and friends. These experiences have all been good ones,' says 24-year-old Bryony, who was brought up by her mum, her mum's female partner and her dad. 'I do feel as though I am part of the LGBT community. It's the world I was brought up in. When I'm supporting gay rights, I feel as though I am supporting something that is a part of me, whether I identify *as LGBT myself or not.'*

'*In my early years, my parents would wheel me around the parade in my buggy,'* remembers Shoshana, also in her early twenties. '*My memories of Pride as a child are bright, colourful and noisy. I remember men dressed in drag with giant multicoloured eyelashes, whistles to blow and horns to beep, glitter, feathers and laughter. I shouldn't downplay the presence of politics either – angry speeches and rousing chants are just as important too. When I was 14, I remember Conservative MP Michael Portillo being booed by an audience still furious about Section 28. But my own sexuality was still a mystery to me then. I was proud of my family and happy to be marching for the LGBT+ community. Now I have a beautiful bunch of LGBT+ friends to walk with. But even if I didn't identify as LGBT+ myself, I'd still like to be there: supporting my family; proudly acknowledging our social significance; and championing LGBT+ visibility and rights.'*

Beyond Pride

While Prides have become increasingly inclusive of lesbians, bi and trans people over the years, this has not always been the case. Women-only or bi- or trans-majority events, organised by and for the community, have been enriching and affirming spaces for parents who hold these identities, including Lea, Miriam, Naomi and Andy/Mina, and their children.

BiCon is a weekend-long educational and social gathering for bi people, their friends, partners, and others with a supportive interest in bisexuality – and Lea loves it. '*BiCon is amazing,'* she enthuses. '*It's important for me to go, so that when my daughter's older she realises she's not the only kid with a parent that doesn't fit into society's norms.'* As a solo parent, having access to a crèche means that Lea can experience the event in her own right, not just as a parent, '*It is wonderful to know I can also make the most of sessions I wish to attend, even if perhaps they aren't suitable for my daughter's tender ears,'* she explains.

Miriam hasn't succeeded in meeting LGBT parents locally, so her annual visit to lesbian arts festival L Fest with her daughter is an important part of her connection to the LGBT community. '*We went to a local lesbian parenting group, but the* children were all younger and we didn't have a huge amount in common,' she says. 'Last year we camped in the family area at L Fest and, since then, have stayed in contact with a couple of families that we met. We're seeing them again this year. It's really nice to meet other lesbian families, and to be at an event that's women-focused.'

Naomi, who is pansexual, and Andy/Mina, who is gender-fluid, have taken their five-year-old son to both their local Pride, and to Sparkle, the annual transgender celebration. At Sparkle, Naomi can share her worries about being out with other parents, and they can learn from each other's experiences. 'I talked to other parents at Sparkle when I was anxious about our son's school knowing,' she says, 'but found out from them that often when people do know, they are not shocked and reactions are positive.' Sparkle is a safe space for Naomi's family to relax and have fun for the weekend, as well as to gain strength and encouragement for the rest of the year.

Naomi's experiences at Pride and Sparkle stand in direct contrast to the fears that her parents expressed when she told them she was taking their grandson along. 'I had huge problems with my parents when we took our son to Pride,' she explains. 'My dad said: "I hope the social workers don't find out, they'll take him away." I showed him the Pride stuff from the social workers' union, I explained that social workers would be there celebrating Pride. My dad is worried that Pride is full of bad people and that being around LGBT people could corrupt our child, but he doesn't really know what Pride is. I wish I could take him along to see it's not what he thinks.'

Even though Pride is now mainstream – many would say too mainstream – with support from institutions like the police, all the main political parties and large corporations, there are still plenty of fears and misconceptions about LGBT events, and their suitability for children. As parents, we make decisions for our children every day – what they wear, eat, watch or do. We do our utmost to ensure they stay safe, happy and can be themselves. That may mean marching as a family at Pride or celebrating at Sparkle; connecting with other LGBT parents online or in the local park; joining campaigns for LGBT equality; or simply hanging out with old and new friends, reminiscing about our child-free days and gossiping about which celebrities have recently come out. There are so many ways for us and our children to be proud, stay gay and nourish our roots within the LGBT community.

Top tips

1. **Look around.** Think about what's most important to you. Is it friendship, visibility, positive role models for your children, maintaining a link to the LGBT community, political action or something else? Look around for a group, event or online network that's the best fit. This may change as your children get older.

2. **Manage your expectations.** In a parent-and-toddler group, you are likely to spend more time complaining about sleep deprivation than discussing queer politics. However much you love Pride, a city-centre march might be too much when toilet-training your two-year-old. You may find LGBT parents going through exactly the same issues as you, or you may feel baffled by other people's struggles and choices and relate better with other parents with whom you have something else in common.

3. **Celebrate diversity.** If you are part of an LGBT parents' group or at an LGBT event, try to make sure that all types of family feel that they are fully welcome. While we may have our differences, we are stronger together.

4. **Do it yourself.** Nothing out there for you? The power of social media means that it's never been easier to set up and advertise your own group. It's even easier with a friend or group of friends, to give you the confidence that it's not going to be just you at the first meeting! Lesbian mum Victoria has set up a local group for LGBT parents – a Facebook page and the occasional Saturday meet-up at the park – because, as she says, *we lead such a straight life, and it's nice to hang out with people who are gay. As our son grows up, he'll see families similar to his. Being a parent is fantastic and rewarding, but every day you are reminded of your difference and that can be hard work. That's why I value meeting up with a group of other gay parents.*

16

NOT IN FRONT OF THE CHILDREN

This chapter covers why, how and when LGBT parents choose to talk with their children about sex and relationships, homophobia, diversity and what it means for them to be part of an LGBT family, helping them to be confident in their own story and in sharing it with others.

This isn't about a single conversation or once-in-a-lifetime moment of truth. It's about chats over breakfast, in the bath, in the car, after someone's said something horrible at school or when you're watching TV together. It's about what we do as families when we tell and retell our own stories to each other: we remind ourselves of the bonds of love we create and share together. That's not an LGBT family thing; it's a family thing.

We need our children to know what makes their family different from others, as well as what makes it the same, so that they can better understand themselves and take their place confidently in the world. But it can be a fine balance, as lesbian mum Mel puts it, *'between telling them enough, without telling them too much'*. And, just when you think you know what you're doing, things change: your children get older and you encounter new questions, challenges and situations. *'It's hard to learn how to be a good parent,'* reflects mother of two Rajo. *'But the children have taught me to be as honest as I can be. I say when I don't know something, when I don't have all the answers. I tell my children, I've never been a parent before, so we're going to have to work this out together as a family.'*

Rajo and her partner have two teenage children and have found that, with each year that goes by, their children have new questions about how they came to create their family. *'When they were about five, we explained that we'd been to hospital to have a special injection of liquid which was mixed with the eggs to make a baby. It was our daughter who asked whether they both had the same liquid.*

'By the time they were six, they understood that there was no blood link between them because they didn't have the same donor. It took a while for them to get their heads round it, but by seven they were saying how cool it was that we got to choose. Then, when they properly understood, they both asked why we didn't choose someone they knew. So then we had to explain about sperm donors, why they do it, why there's a hospital in the middle. At nine, our daughter asked whether she could find her donor if she wanted to. We said we weren't sure how, it would probably be possible but she'd need to think about why she'd want to find out.' Rajo's answers were clear and relevant, not just dealing with biological facts, but also with the emotional impact of what those facts meant for the family. As her children move through adolescence, and even adulthood, one thing is certain – the questions and conversations will continue.

Telling the story

'When you're a non-traditional family you have to be much more upfront, there can't be a veil of secrecy. A child should never find out where they come from, they should always know,' says Evan, who, with his partner, Felix, had their son through surrogacy. Many LGBT parents today would strongly agree – both for practical reasons, and for the emotional well-being of the whole family.

Jenny stresses the importance of talking honestly with your children about their origins. She and her partner had their two children, now four and six years old, via IVF using donor eggs and donor sperm. *'Before we had them, we went to a Donor Conception Network workshop on parenting,'* she remembers. *'The most important thing we learnt was to start telling your child from an early age so that they grow up with it, and they don't remember being sat down and told. They said, "Don't keep any secrets."*

'So from almost before he could understand, we've been telling our son his story. Now, we need to start telling his little sister as well. We've told him that Mummy Jenny and Mummy Lucy wanted to have a baby and couldn't have one, so they went on a plane to another country, and a kind man and kind woman

took a seed and an egg and put it in Mummy Lucy's tummy.

'*It grew and grew and grew and at the end of nine months, who popped out? Then he shouts out his name. And then two years later the same thing happened, it grew and grew and grew and who popped out? And then he shouts his sister's name and says, "I came before her, didn't I?"*' In the telling and retelling, this stops being just Jenny and Lucy's story, it becomes his story too. In fact, he's got the starring role and gets to define what's most important for him right now: not having two mummies, but being the big brother.

The fear often expressed by those opposed to LGBT parenting is that children will be indoctrinated or sexualised from an early age if they learn about LGBT relationships when they are 'too young to understand'. But when we talk with very young children, we're not giving a sex education lesson or a queer theory tutorial, although trying not to confuse our children about matters of human biology is still a good idea! We're telling them a story about how much they are loved, wanted and surrounded by people who care for them.

'*One evening after nursery, my son asked me, "Why don't you and Daddy live together?"*' says Poppy. '*So I explained that we're not together any more and lots of people don't live with both their parents. He asked, "Why do you live with Kelsey and Kelsey's a girl?" I told him it's because Mummy and Kelsey love each other, and that sometimes a girl loves a girl. He said, "Oh, okay," and went back to eating his tea.*'

Poppy's son was much more interested in his fish fingers than in a long discussion about who loves whom, because it's obvious to him that he's part of a loving family. '*My son sees his father every weekend,*' continues Poppy. '*Now my ex's expecting a baby with his fiancée. I think it will be great for my son to have a brother or sister. His father and I don't always agree on parenting. But we're amicable and we both know our son is the most important thing and want to be friends for him.*'

Many families, both LGBT and straight, are like Poppy's, with children part of a web of love and connection that extends beyond their own home. However, sometimes those webs are more complicated in LGBT families than they are in other kinds of families. Explaining them in ways that make sense to young children takes thought and creativity.

Felix and Evan describe their journey of starting a family via surrogacy as '*a concerted team effort and lots of logistics*'. It's important to them that their son knows about the team who created him. '*We made him a book about Daddy Evan and Daddy Felix, with pictures of our surrogate and her family and her bump, the egg donor and her family, and the time when he was born,*' explains Felix. '*The first few times we read it with him it went over his head, but he loved the pictures of himself. He understands more now, and knows that as two men we needed a woman. That book has been great, even before he met our surrogate's children, he knew their names. God knows what he thinks about putting eggs in her tummy though, he really likes eggs.*'

Now that they are planning their second child and, for medical reasons, can't use the same egg donor, they are pondering how best to tell the story this time: '*The key difference is that we have an anonymous egg donor through the clinic. We have pictures of our son's egg donor, but we won't have that for the second child. We just have one sentence about her: that she likes roller hockey and supports her husband. We'll probably major on roller hockey, but I wonder whether one day, when we're all obsessed by roller hockey, we'll find out that she wasn't interested in it at all, it was just something she wrote on the form.*'

Sharing the story

With very young children, there is no sense in telling them something and expecting them to keep it to themselves. All parents – except the superhumanly tactful – have experienced the horror of your small child loudly and innocently repeating remarks which were never meant for a public audience. If you are out to your children, you're out to the world, even if this isn't always what you would choose. '*Being an LGBT parent means always being out, and always having to come out. If I am honest, I am not always comfortable with it, I wish I could be,*' says lesbian mum of two Heather, while simultaneously recognising that if she wants her children to be at ease with themselves and proud of their family, then she needs to model what this looks like. '*I will always tell people who we are to our children, as I will not let them see me deny who we are. But I anticipate that moment before people respond, when I can see that they are thinking what to say, how to sound accepting whether they are or not. I am very conscious of my children not internalising homophobia, as I must have done, so I try to be matter-of-fact about us.'*

Working with our children to find a story that they can share is very important. The words they use to describe their families need to make sense in the context of their friends' families too, even if that means simplifying more complex information.

How do we tell a consistent story, the one that makes sense when our children are toddlers and when they are teenagers? The language has to change to be more age-appropriate, and the fundamentals need to stay the same. Nicki has some good advice, which makes sense whatever age your children are. *'You've got to work as a team, and not expect too much of your children,'* she counsels. *'You can give them information that's true, but relevant for their age, and a story that they can share with other people, but they've got to work things out for themselves. We're there to support their choices. You can't get cross with them for finding their own path.'*

Nicki's son was born with help from a known donor, who was uninvolved in her son's life for many years. She explains the kind of shareable story that he needed as he got older and began to notice his family was different from his friends'. *'When our son asked why he couldn't see his dad, we could tell him that his dad was a kind man who helped us, but we didn't know him very well,'* says Nicki. *'But he could tell people at school that he did have a dad, it's just that his dad didn't live with him, and that's something lots of people say.'*

Like Nicki, Dónal found that his children were taking the information he and his partner had shared with them, and adapting it to answer the questions they encountered at school. *'As a family, we tend to chat in the car. The boys seem to find it less challenging,'* he explains. *'Many of those chats have been about our family make-up. The boys seem to get that they had a mum and a dad who couldn't keep them safe, so they moved in with their foster carers until their forever family was found. A few months in, our youngest came home from school and said that a girl in his class said that everyone has a mummy, so he couldn't have two dads. Without batting an eyelid, he'd responded that he has a mum, but she was a bit rubbish (not my words) so now he has two dads.'*

Although Nicki's son doesn't live with his biological dad, he still says he's got a dad, and although Dónal's sons don't live with their birth mother, they still say they've got a mum. For many LGBT parents, this isn't the case. They too will have to consider honest and appropriate answers to the same question as their children grow up. Some choose to focus the story on what their children *do* have, rather than what they *don't*. *'I don't know when the children are going to start asking more about dads,'* says lesbian mum Jenny. *'They have an awareness that other people have dads. Occasionally our son, who's six now, has said, "I'd like a dad." While we validate his feelings, we also try to point out the positives. It's like, "well, you've got two mums, not a lot of people have two mums"'.*

Shoshana was brought up by her mums, and remembers at school having to explain and justify why she didn't have a dad. *'We were studying the life cycle of a frog and the teacher referenced the role of mummies and daddies,'* she recalls. *'During the ensuing conversation, little me piped up, "I don't have a daddy; I have a sperm donor." This was immediately rubbished by the teacher, who told me that of course I had a daddy – everybody has a daddy. She explained that her little girl didn't see her daddy, but she still had one, and so did I. I went home perplexed and recounted this to my parents. They decided to talk to the school – it's not okay for a teacher to critique a little girl's sense of self. The school backed my parents up. And I went home the next day happy in the knowledge that while the teacher's little girl might have a daddy, I didn't, and that both situations were perfect for both little girls.'*

Jim and Katie are open with their sons about their father's gender identity, and the fact they were donor-conceived: *'We decided that we would talk to them about Jim's identity from an early age. We framed it as "when Daddy was little, everyone thought he was a girl – but inside, he knew he was a boy"'.*

However, it was trickier to help their sons understand that this wasn't something to be shared with everyone. *'We've taken the approach that it's not a secret, but it is private,'* says Katie. *'That puts it in the same box as other things which we are quite open about within the family, but encourage them not to share widely, for example, we don't have many family taboos around nakedness, or talking about our bodies. There have been a couple of occasions when one of them announced to the world in general, "My daddy used to be a girl." I've tried to gently acknowledge what they were saying, remind them that it's a private thing, and encourage the conversation onto other ground.'*

Sophie and her partner co-parent their daughter with a known donor. She's only eight months old, so a little young for discussions about her conception and parentage. But they know that questions will come, because they already get these questions themselves. *'When people ask questions, we know that really they want to know the nitty-gritty details: did we use a clinic, was there sex involved, or was it a DIY job? To us, this is unacceptable. You don't ask straight couples what kind of sex they had that night, or what position, or how many times they did it,'* states Sophie firmly.

That's why she and her partner agreed that only themselves and their child will know the details. Sophie continues, *'If people ask, we simply explain that we co-parent. If people push for more we say that, just like any other child, a sperm and an egg created her. As we bring up our daughter, we hope to instil in her a sense that, although on the surface people may see a difference, at the core her family is no different: she has parents who take care of her and love her; she has a safe, stable home; she is happy and healthy.'*

Let's talk about sex

LGBT parents have a double task to face: educating our children both about how babies are made, and about sex. In many books and in much sex education for children, or even teenagers, the two are conflated: sex is what you do to have babies; babies are born as a result of sex. But we know that neither of those are necessarily the case.

You can't just sit back and wait for school. Miriam, a lesbian mum and a secondary school biology teacher, explains that, from her experience, *'at school, they only learn about heterosexual sex, and not much beyond reproduction. What they get for sex education at school is so perfunctory, so heteronormative. These kids have no idea about how you can or can't get pregnant, no idea about their own anatomy and their bodies, nothing about gay or lesbian sex at all.'*

So what to do? Being as clear and upfront as possible, and being prepared to answer questions as they come up, has worked well so far for Jessica and her partner, as it has for many other LGBT parents. They conceived their two daughters with sperm from Simon, a close and long-standing friend of Jessica's. *'We've always explained everything with the correct biological terms,'* Jessica says. *'Once I overheard my partner talking with the girls about sperm and eggs and testicles, and that to make babies a man might put his penis in a woman. Then there was a pause, "But Mummy and Simon didn't do that, did they?" asked our daughter. So we explained, it can happen that way, but there are other ways too. They have a very good understanding of biological process. Most importantly, they know that we chose to create them.'*

'Talking about sex is one of the things we are beginning to have to deal with,' adds Katie who is married to Jim with eight- and 11-year-old sons. *'We've been pretty open with them and tried to answer their questions about where babies come from as honestly as we can. The penny has just dropped with our elder son that our sex life is probably not what he has been taught at school. We don't think we should share with him what we do in bed – no one likes their parents talking about sex – but somehow we have to help him understand that we have a rich and fulfilling sexual relationship without a fully functioning penis. I suspect this will be a challenge to a teenage boy!'*

Unlike Jim, who transitioned before his children were born, Susie is in the process of transitioning just as her children are entering adolescence. There are hormones raging on all sides. *'I get "woman questions" from my daughter now, as she's closer to me than she is to her biological mother,'* says Susie, slightly bemused. *'When her periods started, she was asking me questions. I had to tell her, "I'm not qualified to help with that, I haven't got the right bits, you need to ask your bio mum about this."*

'She's also said, "If you're growing boobs and getting spots, does that mean you're going through puberty like me?" I said, "I suppose I am." But I have to be careful: she's not my sister, she's

my daughter and she needs to grow up at her own pace.'

It's not easy to find the happy medium between skirting round an issue and giving too much information. Sometimes we'll get it right and can congratulate ourselves on our superb parenting skills. Sometimes we'll get it wrong and discover later that we've upset or confused our children. However, if we keep talking, there's always another chance to get it right, to clarify what you meant, to use different language, answer questions in another way or have the conversation at a better time.

Just keep talking, that's Cathy's advice. She's been there, done that, and is now doing it all again. She came out and separated from her husband when their four children were all at primary school; now they are adults with their own families, and she and her female partner are bringing up their 11-year-old granddaughter. They've been though plenty of ups and downs, but her advice stays the same, whatever the circumstances: *'Just be yourself. Be proud of who you are. Don't ever hide it,'* she says. *'Talk to your children. If they've got any questions, then be open with them. Keep talking to each other, that's the main thing.'*

'It's so gay': Helping your children deal with homophobia

Telling your children that they are loved and wanted is the easy bit. Talking about sperm and eggs and sex and birth, even for those of us who are more uptight and inhibited, isn't that bad either. What is much harder is helping your children to face homophobia, transphobia, bullying and exclusion of LGBT people and their families.

There are times when your role as a parent is to protect, rather than explain, to show your children by your response how they too can deal with adversity. Mel knows what it's like to go through tough times simply for being an LGBT family. *'We've moved twice because of the abuse,'* she says. *'We had graffiti sprayed on our wall, saying we were scum, and we had faeces through the door. There were some really dark days. Just me and two little people depending on me, so I've had to be strong. I never would have imagined the things that the girls and I have been through in the last two years, but we have come through and we are a strong family unit. It's getting better now.'*

While extreme prejudice clearly does exist, as Mel's family know more than anyone should have to, casual ridiculing of people who are different is more common. Celebrating diversity and being proud and upfront about being LGBT helps children to be confident in themselves too – in particular by using the word 'gay' in a positive, descriptive way, before they start hearing it used as a playground term of abuse. *'I heard my daughter playing outside with some kids, and one of them was using "gay" to insult another kid,'* says lesbian mum Chantelle, whose daughter is eight. *'She had no idea what he was talking about. "Gay" isn't a bad thing to her; it's just a thing. She knows Mummy loves Linda, and Grandma loves Granddad, people love whoever they love.'* This, then, helps her to articulate and explore her own feelings. Chantelle continues, *'At the moment, when she grows up she wants to marry my partner's daughter, who she's really close to, but she's also got a "boyfriend" in her class. She knows it's not who they are, but how she feels with that person, that matters.'*

Susie has been honest with her two children about her transition, keeping communication open, without forcing any issues that her children are not ready for: *'I've said to them I won't talk about it unless you want me to, but nothing is off limits if you do.'* This means that, rather than silently worrying, they have been able to bring their fears to her: *'My son worries about my safety, he warns me not to get beaten up. I've only ever been attacked once, and that caused him a lot of sadness.'* Despite her upbeat attitude, Susie knows that you can't pretend bad things won't happen, even if they are rare. But by keeping them in perspective and maintaining open and honest communication, she believes you can make it less likely that your children will try to deal with their fears alone.

As his sons are getting older, Dónal is coming to terms with the same challenge. *'Our boys are old enough to understand that being gay is not the norm,'* he says of his two sons, aged eight and nine. *'They are resilient lads and will be able to deal with teasing. Our job now is to convince them that they can talk to us. We do not need them to protect us. We need to know if they are being bullied for any reason, including homophobia. As they approach their teens, it's likely that they will go through periods of wanting to fit in, so are likely to push us away when they are with friends. I'm going to find this difficult, but have to remind myself that this too will pass.'*

Well before adolescence, children become aware of difference and the pressure to fit in. This can manifest itself as embarrassment about their family (something that every child in every type of family experiences at some point) or even as homophobic behaviour. Knowing where to set limits and when to allow your children time to work things out for themselves is not an easy decision, as lesbian mums Rosie and Nicki found out. *'When our son was eight or nine, things became difficult,'* says Rosie. *'When we went on holiday, he said that he was going to call me "aunty" instead of "mummy". We said to him, you can say what you want. But of course he kept forgetting and calling me "mummy" anyway.'*

'Then he went through a homophobic period,' adds Rosie's partner, Nicki. *'He said really horrible things to us. Once Rosie was so upset that she left the house. When she came back, he said, "Sorry, Mum, for dissing your culture." That was the turning point, him seeing how upset she got.'*

There are things we can do about homophobia and transphobia. We can join campaigns, we can challenge offensive comments that we overhear and we can become visible role models, showing that being LGBT is nothing to be ashamed or afraid of. *'There's so much misinformation out there about gay parents,'* says lesbian mum of two Jessica. *'So every year I go and talk to a local LGBT youth group about being a lesbian parent. I think it's important for them to hear from an ancient person like me about how having children is just a normal part of my life.'*

There are times when it is not safe to be outspoken but, for many of us, direct experience of prejudice is unusual. *'I get a shock when I hear something negative said about gay or lesbian parents,'* continues Jessica. *'I do a double take – first of all, I'm shocked because it's so unkind, and then a second later I realise, oh my goodness, they are talking about me and my family. It's a terrible reminder that prejudice is still out there.'* These are the times when it's more important to stand out rather than blend in, showing our children that prejudice against anyone for any reason is not acceptable. The courage and conviction to stand up against injustice, whether or not it is targeted directly at us, is one of the most important parenting lessons we can give.

Understanding the past

In the UK today, children can see same-sex couples getting married, and celebrities who come out or transition being applauded for their honesty. They can see LGBT people in the public eye as politicians and opinion-formers, and when anti-gay comments are reported in the media or overheard in conversation, they are frequently challenged or condemned, rather than endorsed.

It's very different from when Gill brought up her son in a lesbian household in the 1970s. While she was out as a lesbian in feminist circles, it would have been risky for her to be more open about her sexuality. Lesbian parents were regarded with suspicion and custody rulings invariably went against them simply because of their sexual orientation. So Gill publicly identified as a single mother out of a desire to safeguard her family. Her concern was always to both protect her son and be as honest with him as possible. Not always an easy balance to strike.

'My policy from the beginning (having no role models or knowledge to work from) was to tell no lies and to answer any questions as honestly as possible,' explains Gill. 'As my son grew up, he had his first girlfriends and was clearly heterosexual. We discussed sex, sexuality, and relationships, as matters came up; I always said to him that I had my own strong opinions, and would tell him what they were if he asked, but that he should always form his own views.' However, there were times when she encouraged him to be discreet about his family at school or with friends, simply because 'I wanted to protect him from inheriting prejudice and bigotry, when I could'.

Many LGBT parents bringing up children today will have experienced some kind of prejudice. We may have grown up surrounded by negative attitudes about LGBT people and with few positive role models. It's likely we have internalised some of the beliefs we encountered at an early age, however much we try to shake them off now. Shirley and Ailsa, parents of twin boys, recognise that they carry their childhood experiences with them into adulthood. They admit that even today *'we both fear prejudice and we don't want the boys to suffer. Ailsa's experience of school was extreme homophobia and she became homophobic herself in order to fit in. Shirley grew up in a socially liberal family, but still remembers homophobia in the playground.'*

Even events that happened decades ago can have an impact on families today. It may be necessary to share the past with children in appropriate ways. Jim and Katie have found this a painful issue to address with their two sons, but ultimately could not avoid it. Katie explains, *'For a long time, the one thing we hadn't shared with the boys was how tough life had been for Jim as a young person. When he was growing up in the 1960s and 70s, trans people were viewed as weird aberrations, probably psychologically imbalanced and definitely misguided. The leading gender clinic in the country told Jim's parents that it was "just a phase". In his late teens, Jim was sent to a psychiatric unit and subjected to repeated ECT treatment – which left him with severe and lifelong memory problems. This and other experiences of rejection and stigmatisation have left Jim emotionally vulnerable.*

'On one occasion, Jim and I had an argument just after the boys had gone to bed, which ended with us both shouting, and him swearing loudly and leaving the house. Our older son was distraught, worried that Jim and I were going to split up, and frightened. Our younger son, who is much less able to talk about his feelings, was just very quiet.

'I felt I had to explain where some of this had come from, and why Dad had lost his temper, so I talked to them about some of the things that had happened to him. We all cried and, when Jim came back in, we had some hugs and more tears. These moments, which afterwards seem significant milestones, always take you unawares – which means you end up muddling through as best you can at the time.'

A complex web of experiences and identities shape us as we grow up, and they can't always be neatly separated out into cause and effect. When Jackie was bringing up her son, Jacob, and her partner's son as a single parent in the 1990s, there were few role models for lesbian parents and she was unsure herself whether to identify as lesbian or bisexual. This contributed to her decision not to come out to Jacob until he was a teenager, but also she recognises that fear was a driving force behind the decision.

'I think being a Jewish lesbian has complications,' she reflects, years later. 'I'm also the daughter of a Holocaust survivor. So there is terror ingrained within the marrow of my bones. I was mistakenly trying to protect them and myself, because I was under an illusion that bad things would happen if I came out. I don't think they would have done, but that was my fear at the time.

'Something happened, it might have been that the fear reduced, it might have been social changes, but then I thought I could come out. Once Jacob got over his initial upset and anger that I hadn't been honest with him, he was so proud. By the time he was 20, he could say, "I now totally get why you did it, I don't blame you."'

Today, Jacob remembers how and when he started to realise that his mum was a lesbian, and the impact that realisation had on him as a teenager becoming aware of his own sexuality. 'My mum never properly came out to me. I found out about her sexuality from overhearing conversations and piecing things together,' he recalls. 'I hate to say that my initial reaction was shame. Even though I was not straight myself, I was closeted at that time and still harbouring lots of internalised hatred. It wasn't until I confronted my mother about her sexuality that we finally had a conversation about it. I had initially felt betrayed and her first response was that this was her information to share or not share. While this is true, I still felt that it was also part of my story. This is something that we have both since come to understand. I now appreciate that the real culprit in her decision to keep the secret from me is homophobia in our society. Still, it's much harder to be angry at a system of oppression than a person.

'My subsequent coming out at the age of nineteen meant that both of us were able to live open and honest lives, something I treasure. My understanding of my own family has developed over time and, while it can be a complicated story to tell, I am proud to speak with people about my unique family background.'

Looking back and understanding the past – our own, our family's and our society's – helps us understand the people we are now and reflect on the decisions we make. It also reminds us how times have changed. Not just in terms of how open we are with our children about sexual orientation or growing up in an LGBT family, but how open we are with our children in every way. Jackie's unshockable, unstoppable 95-year-old aunt Leila helps put it into perspective. *'I like the way it is more open today. The attitude when I was growing up was so different,'* she says, explaining that *'when I had my first period at 11, I had no idea what was happening. My mum slapped me round the face, and said; "Now you're a woman." When my younger brother was born I was seven, my parents told me they'd found him under a tree. Today, there are so many married couples who separate and divorce, so many children who don't have a dad because he's gone away or died, so it's not just in lesbian families that a child doesn't have a dad. There are lots of different families. If children know where they come from, they grow up more open-minded.'*

Acknowledging difference, celebrating diversity
When you're a kid, your family is normal because it's your family. It's also weird and embarrassing because it's your family, regardless of whether your parents are LGBT or not.

Shoshana is biracial, Jewish and was brought up by her two mums. Although people would notice and comment on this throughout her childhood, it wasn't always these things that they noticed: *'At a post-party sleepover, aged 16, I was talking with a girl in my year group whom I'd never been particularly close to,'* she remembers. *'She said the only thing she knew about my family was that we scraped the butter rather than dug at it (really? Is that gossip worthy?). Yet somehow I'd imagined that my situation was prime gossip, and that the news got around.'*

There can be a certain cachet about being different. *'Our girls are very open about their family,'* says Jessica. *'There have been times when we've been camping, they've been out playing with other children on the campsite, and have come back to the tent, pointed to us drinking tea and reading the paper and said, "See, I told you so," to their new friends.'*

For many children in LGBT families, their family set-up is a non-issue except when they get asked questions about it. So many of the questions addressed in this chapter – what to tell and when and how – are things that parents worry about, but are of little interest to their children. *'I've always known my mums are gay, they hug and kiss so I've always known,'* says 11-year-old Milly, as if she's been asked a ridiculous question. *'I haven't needed any books about gay families, my mums just explained. They didn't sit me down seriously, I always knew. If friends ask, I explain, but I don't say anything if they don't ask.'*

Yes, we need to prepare our children that their family might be different from their friends' families. Yes, we need to help them articulate why it's different and to take pride in it, as well as help them notice similarities and areas of common ground. Yes, we need to give them the tools to cope with any homophobia or transphobia they encounter. But the most positive message we can give them is one which *all* children need to hear and own, not just children in LGBT families: diversity is good and our differences enrich us all. Not an easy message to believe, particularly during the teenage years with their pressure to conform, but a crucial one.

Rajo explains it to her children like this: *'I say to them, no two people have the same fingerprint or DNA, so why worry about being different? We're all created different for a reason.'* But she recognises that explanations from her can only go so far. *'Looking back, we probably should have been more proactive at mixing with LGBT and different families. I'd like them to have other teenagers to talk to from LGBT families, and form honest friendships where they can compare experiences. I don't know what it's like to be a teenager now, so they need to talk to their peers who are also in different family set-ups. We talk about different families, but actually meeting them reinforces that different is good.'*

Looking back on her childhood, Shoshana cannot remember a *'moment when I realised I was different for having two mums. I always knew because I was always brought up being told and, more importantly, shown so.'* She was brought up to understand that relationships are diverse and wonderful. She continues, *'I grew up easy in the knowledge that some women like men and some women like women and some men like men, and some people like both genders. And that when I grew up I could love whoever I wanted to love. It would be fantastic if that was a message we could give to all of our children.'*

Chantelle laughs about all the ways that people might label her as different. *'There's a running joke in our house that we fit all the minorities: Greek, disabled, single parent, gay – just pile them all on!'* she says. *'When I do something shocking, people who know me say, "That's such a Chantelle thing to do, classic Chan." But I think being normal is beige and dull. I want my daughter to brightly stand out, to reflect luminous and not to be afraid of who she wants to be.'*

Whatever their family shape, size or structure, whatever their ethnicity, religion or colour, surely that's what we all want for our children: a chance for them to shine brightly, love richly and to be whoever they want to be.

Top tips

1. **Start young.** Even if you are not visible as an LGBT family and there's no external pressure to be out, it's still important not to keep secrets within the family. Otherwise, if you are only honest with your children once they are older, being part of an LGBT family risks being a much bigger deal than it needs to be.

2. **Keep talking.** It's likely you will have many conversations with your children about the issues in this chapter as they grow older. New experiences will mean new questions. You won't always have the right words or know all the answers, but you can be ready to listen, learn and work it out together.

3. **It's okay to be discreet.** You don't have to talk about everything with everyone, all the time. This is your story as much as it your children's. Many parents have found it helpful to teach their children the distinction between secret – something perceived as hidden and shameful – and private – something which is perfectly okay but not necessarily for public sharing.

4. **Look for resources.** There are a growing number of children's books that touch on LGBT families, although they are mostly for young children rather than teenagers or older primary school children. Reading them aloud and

having them on the shelf gives you something to explore together and refer back to later. Discussing TV programmes, films, news stories and other people's families (although preferably not right in front of them) can also open up conversations about diversity and difference.

Acknowledgments

Our greatest thanks go to all the LGBT parents, children from LGBT families and friends of LGBT families who shared their experiences with us. Your stories and wisdom are at the heart of this book and *Pride and Joy* would not exist without you. Thank you for taking the time to be interviewed or to email us answers to questions or previously written articles, and for being so honest and generous in your responses. We've been inspired and encouraged by hearing your stories, and we're delighted to be able to share them through these pages.

We gathered enough material to fill ten books, and regrettably we couldn't include everyone's contribution. But every submission, interview or conversation has influenced and informed *Pride and Joy*, whether or not you were directly quoted – so thank you to all who contributed their stories. Special thanks to everyone in the *Pride and Joy* Facebook group who answered our random questions, offered good advice and encouraged us to keep going.

We found contributors through friends, colleagues, family members, and LGBT networks (Stonewall in particular and many others too). But soon *Pride and Joy* took on a life of its own, and we started getting emails every day from people wanting to take part. Special thanks to those contributors who took on the challenge of helping us find other contributors, in particular Justine Smithies, Nicki Stott and Heather Liveston.

Thank you to those people who helped us to turn a rough-and-ready manuscript into a coherent story: Sophie Parker-Manuel, Jess Monck, Scott Casson-Rennie, Ric and Craig, Nicki Stott and Ramona Franklyn for reading and commenting on early chapters; Gideon Burrows and Christine Smith for advice on getting published; Emma Grundy Haigh, our editor, for incisive comments and questions; and Martin Wagner, Zoë Blanc, Zoë Hutton and all at Pinter & Martin for believing in *Pride and Joy* and for getting as excited as we are about this book.

Thank you to Helen Bilton for introducing us to Pinter & Martin and for your indexing skills, and thanks to Emma Frith for coming up with the inspired title – *Pride and Joy*.

Thank you to our own families, Mary and Alan Hagger and Chris, Vivien and Laurie Holt, for your love and care as we grew up, and for the support you've given us as we've become parents. Thank you to Alex Huzzey and David Warren, for embarking on this extraordinary co-parenting journey with us, for your ongoing friendship, and for putting up with us spending a whole holiday hunched over our laptops working on final edits. Thank you to our children, Esther and Miriam, for your enthusiastic ideas on content and publicity, and for not complaining about all the time we spent writing.

Thank you to everyone who has bought and read this book. We are sharing the profits from sales of *Pride and Joy* with organisations providing legal, psychological or practical assistance to LGBT asylum seekers and refugees as they deal with trauma, discrimination and settling into the UK. Thank you for enabling us to support this work.

And finally, thank you to everyone who has encouraged us and told us why you think a book like *Pride and Joy* is really necessary. To everyone who said, after we finished writing our first book *Living It Out*, 'When's your next book coming out?', well, eight years later, here it is.

Index